Endocrinology

TERTIARY LEVEL BIOLOGY

A series covering selected areas of biology at advanced undergraduate level. While designed specifically for course options at this level within Universities and Polytechnics, the series will be of great value to specialists and research workers in other fields who require a knowledge of the essentials of a subject.

Titles in the series:

Experimentation in Biology	Ridgman
Methods in Experimental Biology	Ralph
Visceral Muscle	Huddart and Hunt
Biological Membranes	Harrison and Lunt
Comparative Immunobiology	Manning and Turner
Water and Plants	Meidner and Sheriff
Biology of Nematodes	Croll and Matthews
An Introduction to Biological Rhythms	Saunders
Biology of Ageing	Lamb
Biology of Reproduction	Hogarth
An Introduction to Marine Science	Meadows and Campbell
Biology of Fresh Waters	Maitland
An Introduction to Developmental Biology	Ede
Physiology of Parasites	Chappell
Neurosecretion	Maddrell and Nordmann
Biology of Communication	Lewis and Gower
Population Genetics	Gale
Structure and Biochemistry of Cell Organelles	Reid
Developmental Microbiology	Peberdy
Genetics of Microbes	Bainbridge
Biological Functions of Carbohydrates	Candy

TERTIARY LEVEL BIOLOGY

Endocrinology

GRAHAM J. GOLDSWORTHY, Ph.D.

Reader in Comparative Endocrinology
University of Hull

JOHN ROBINSON, Ph.D.

Lecturer in Zoology
University of Hull

and

WILLIAM MORDUE, D.Sc.

Professor of Zoology
University of Aberdeen

A HALSTED PRESS BOOK

John Wiley and Sons

New York–Toronto

Blackie & Son Limited
Bishopbriggs
Glasgow G64 2NZ

Furnival House
14–18 High Holborn
London WC1V 6BX

Library of Congress Cataloging in Publication Data

Goldsworthy, Graham J.
  Endocrinology.

  "A Halsted Press book."
  1. Endocrinology. 2. Endocrinology, Comparative.
I. Robinson, John, joint author. II. Mordue, W.,
joint author. III. Title. [DNLM: 1. Endocrine
glands. 2. Hormones. WK100 G236e]
QP187.G583   591.1'42   80-18704
ISBN 0-470-27034-9

Filmset by Advanced Filmsetters (Glasgow) Ltd.

Printed in Great Britain by
Thomson Litho Ltd, East Kilbride, Scotland

Preface

ENDOCRINOLOGY BEGAN AS A BRANCH OF MEDICINE—THE STUDY OF THE "ductless glands" and their "internal secretions"—and has grown rapidly as new endocrine tissues have been discovered in a wide variety of animals. Textbooks of endocrinology often reflect this origin, dealing with the subject organ by organ, chapter by chapter. This apparently natural approach is in fact artificial, and tends to emphasize to the student differences in detail that exist between endocrine systems while obscuring their common features; it is assumed that the student will recognize the basic similarities. In writing this book we have attempted to redress this imbalance, taking as our major theme fundamental concepts in endocrinology: endocrine involvement in coordination and control systems; the structure and functioning of endocrine cells; endocrine activity—what affects it and how it can be assessed; and the mechanisms of hormone action at the sub-cellular level. This conceptual framework is given substance throughout the text by reference to appropriate examples. In later chapters, the involvement of hormones in a limited number of specific systems is discussed in detail. We have tried to avoid vague statements and generalizations, but areas of uncertainty and debate have been highlighted to give the student a critical insight into modern aspects of endocrine research.

Examples have been chosen from the whole animal kingdom to illustrate fundamental principles. In this way, the text provides a suitable introduction to advanced studies in vertebrate, invertebrate and comparative endocrinology.

G.J.G.

J.R.

W.M.

v

Acknowledgements

WE THANK OUR MANY COLLEAGUES WHO HAVE HELPED IN THE PREPARATION of this book. In particular we would like to mention Dr Ann Brown, Ms Sue Russell, Mr Colin Wheeler and Mr Huw Davies for their careful reading of the manuscript and helpful suggestions, and Ms Chrissie Ware and Ms Margaret Bowen for their speedy typing of the final draft. Finally, we are indebted to Mr Roland Wheeler-Osman for his patience, tireless effort and inspiration in transforming our vague sketches into the final illustrations. To all of them we gratefully acknowledge our debt.

Contents

A GLOSSARY OF HORMONES AND TERMS

The entries for *hormones* are arranged in this sequence: Chemical nature; site of production and release: Target organ(s); response.

ACTH: see Adrenocorticotropin.

ADH: see Vasopressin.

Adipokinetic Hormone (AKH): Neurosecretory decapeptide of known sequence; from corpus cardiacum of insects: Fat body and flight muscles; lipid metabolism.

Adrenalin/Noradrenalin: Catecholamines (see figure 2.13); from adrenal medulla (chromaffin tissue) and sympathetic nervous system: Tissue metabolism, constriction/relaxation of smooth muscle.

β-adrenergic receptors (β-receptors): Plasma membrane receptors for catecholamines; present in diverse tissues and associated with cAMP-mediated responses.

Adrenocorticoid: Steroid produced in the adrenal cortex.

Adrenocorticotropin (ACTH; Corticotropin): Peptide of known sequence—39 amino acid residues in mammals; from anterior pituitary: Adrenal cortex; synthesis and release of corticosteroids (but not aldosterone; see Renin-Angiotensin).

AKH: see Adipokinetic Hormone.

Aldosterone: Steroid (see figure 2.10); from adrenal cortex: Na^+/K^+ balance in kidney, and amphibian skin.

Androgens: Steroids (see figure 2.9); mainly testicular but also from adrenal: Most tissues; development and maintenance of masculine characteristics, behaviour and physiology (see figures 7.6, 7.7).

Angiotensins: Peptides of known composition (mammals); formed by action of converting enzyme by cleavage of Angiotensin I: Vasoconstriction and release of aldosterone; may control drinking behaviour in some vertebrates.

Annelid Brain Hormone (Regeneration Hormone; Vitellogenic Hormone; Maturation Inhibiting Hormone): Neurosecretion of unknown composition; from brain-infracerebral complex of polychaetes: Regeneration, yolk synthesis and oocyte development.

Antidiuretic Hormone: see Vasopressin.

Brain Hormone, Activation Hormone (AH) or *Ecdysiotropin*: Insect protein of unknown composition; from cerebral neurosecretory cells: Prothoracic gland; stimulates ecdysteroid production.

Bursicon: Insect polypeptide of unknown composition ($c.$ 40×10^3 molecular weight); from neurosecretory cells of brain or ventral nerve cord: Haemocytes; tyrosine metabolism stimulated for tanning of cuticle.

Calcitonin: Peptide of known composition—32 amino acid residues; from "C" cells of thyroid in mammals and ultimobranchial bodies in non-mammalian vertebrates: Skeleton; decreases blood calcium levels.

CDC: Caudo-dorsal neurosecretory cells of the cerebral ganglia in *Lymnaea* (see figure 7.17).

Cholecystokinin: Polypeptide single chain of 33 amino acid residues; from duodenal mucosa: Stimulates enzyme release from exocrine pancreas and bile release from the gall bladder.

Corticosteroids (Cortisol, corticosterone, etc.): Steroids (see figure 2.10); from adrenal cortex: Lipolysis, protein catabolism, gluconeogenesis, osmoregulation (lower vertebrates mainly)

CRF: Corticotropin releasing factor—see Releasing Factors.

Diuretic Hormones (Insect): Polypeptides of unknown composition; neurosecretory origin: Malpighian tubule; increase urine production.

Ecdysone, Ecdysteroid, Moulting Hormone (MH): Insect steroids (see figure 2.11); from prothoracic glands: Epidermis; moulting. Also produced in insect ovary.

Follicle Stimulating Hormone (FSH): Glycoprotein of known composition; from anterior pituitary: Ovarian follicle cells, seminiferous tubules; maturation of gametes (indirectly).

FSH: see Follicle Stimulating Hormone.

Gastrin: Polypeptide single chain of 17 amino acid residues (mammals); from pyloric mucosa: Stimulates secretion of hydrochloric acid in the stomach.

GFR: Glomerular filtration rate.

GIP: see Glucose-dependent Insulin-releasing Peptide.

Glucagon: Polypeptide single chain of 29 amino acid residues; from pancreatic α-cells— Enteroglucagon (structurally different) from intestine: Liver and adipose tissue; hyperglycaemic and hyperlipaemic activity, although response variable throughout vertebrates.

Glucocorticoid: Adrenocortical steroids which affect intermediary metabolism.

Glucose-dependent Insulin-releasing Peptide (GIP): Polypeptide (see figure 5.2); from intestine: Inhibits gastric secretion, releases insulin.

Gn-RH: see Gonadotropin-releasing Hormone.

Gonadotropin-releasing Hormone (Gn-RH): decapeptide (see figure 7.3); from hypothalamus: anterior pituitary; synthesis and release of FSH and LH.

Growth Hormone (GH, Somatotropin): Vertebrate protein of known composition—about 190 amino acid residues; from anterior pituitary: All tissues; metabolic effects such as protein synthesis, lipolysis, bone deposition.

Growth Hormone (Molluscan): Of unknown nature; from neurosecretory cells (LGC) in cerebral ganglia: Probably the mantle; increases shell growth, but acts on other tissues too.

(Human) Chorionic Gonadotropin (HCG): Glycoprotein of known composition—about 190 amino acid residues; from trophoblast of placenta (i.e. embryonic): Maintenance of corpus luteum.

Hyperglycaemic Hormones (Insects and Crustacea): Polypeptides of unknown composition; neurosecretory origin: Fat body/hepatopancreas; glycogenolysis.

Hypophysectomy: Surgical removal of the pituitary.

Insulin: Polypeptide of known composition (see figure 2.5); from pancreatic β-cells: Most tissues; metabolic regulation and entry of glucose in most tissues (not liver)—hypoglycaemic, hypolipaemic.

Juvenile Hormones: Insect terpenoids (see figure 2.12); from corpora allata; Epidermal and ovarian tissue; metamorphosis and reproduction.

LGC: Light green neurosecretory cells of the cerebral ganglia in *Lymnaea* (see figure 7.17).

LH: see Luteinizing Hormone.

β-lipotropin: Large polypeptide of known composition (see figure 2.8); from anterior pituitary: Hyperlipaemic activity, but physiological significance uncertain.

Luteinizing Hormone (LH) or *Interstitial Cell Stimulating Hormone* (ICSH): Glycoprotein of known composition; from anterior pituitary: Ovary and testis; synthesis of gonadal hormones (oestrogens, progesterone and androgens), ovulation.

Luteolysin: Identified as $PGF_2\alpha$ in several mammals; from uterine endometrium: Termination of corpus luteum steroidogenesis.

Luteotropic Hormone: see Prolactin.

Melanocyte Stimulating Hormone (MSH): Polypeptide with many polymorphic forms (see figure 2.8); from intermediate lobe of pituitary: Dispersal of melanin in melanocytes.

Melatonin: A derivative of 5-hydroxytryptamine; from pineal gland: Hypothalamus; may regulate release of pituitary hormones.

Mineralocorticoid: Adrenocortical steroids which affect ionic regulation.

Moult Inhibiting Hormone: Crustacean protein of unknown composition; from neurosecretory cells in X-organ: Y-organ; prevents ecdysteroid production.

Moulting Hormone: see Ecdysteroids.

MSH: see Melanocyte-Stimulating Hormone.

Neurohypophysial Peptides: Hormones from the posterior pituitary.

Oestrogens: Steroids (see figure 2.9); mainly ovarian but also placental and adrenal origin: Most tissues; development and maintenance of feminine characteristics, behaviour and physiology.

Ovulation Hormone (Molluscan): Peptides of unknown composition; neurosecretory in origin but sites vary according to species: Ovotestis; ovulation, packaging of eggs and egg laying behaviour.

Oxytocin: Octapeptide (see figure 1.3); from hypothalamic neurosecretory cells: Contraction of uterus and "milk let-down" from mammary glands.

Parathormone: see Parathyroid Hormone.

Parathyroid Hormone (PTH): Peptide of known composition—84 amino acid residues; from parathyroids: Skeleton and kidneys; elevates blood calcium levels.

PR-IH: Prolactin Release-inhibiting Hormone: see Releasing Factors.

Progesterone: Steroid (see figure 2.9); from corpus luteum and placenta: Uterus and mammary glands; maintenance of pregnancy, growth of mammary glands.

Prolactin or *Luteotropic Hormone* (LTH): Proteins of known composition—about 190 amino acid residues; from anterior pituitary: Mammary glands, pigeon crop glands, other tissues; milk production, osmoregulation in fish, growth of amphibian tadpoles, maintenance of corpus luteum.

Prostaglandins (PGF$_2\alpha$ etc.): 20-carbon unsaturated fatty acids (see figure 2.14); ubiquitous: Most tissues; diverse effects.

PTH: see Parathyroid Hormone.

Releasing Factors (Releasing Hormones and Release-inhibiting Hormones): Presumed to be peptides but only 3 of established composition—TRH (thyroid stimulating hormone releasing hormone), Somatostatin (growth hormone release-inhibiting hormone) and Gn-RH (gonadotropin releasing hormone); mainly from hypothalamus (but see figure 1.2): Control of release of anterior pituitary hormones.

Renin: Enzyme; from juxtaglomerular cells: Catalyses the conversion of a blood plasma globulin, angiotensinogen, to decapeptide angiotensin I.

Secretin: Polypeptide (see figure 5.2); from upper intestine: Stimulates bicarbonate secretion of pancreas and biliary tract.

Shedding Hormone (Echinoderms): Peptides of unknown composition (c. 2200 molecular weight), species differences known; from radial nerves: Follicle cells of gonads; production of 1-methyladenine to induce maturation of the oocytes.

Somatomedins: Small polypeptides (A and B) of known composition; from liver in response to growth hormone: Action *in vivo* uncertain but have growth-promoting and some insulin-like activity.

Somatostatin: see Releasing Factors.

T$_3$, T$_4$: see Thyronines.

Thyroid Stimulating Hormone (TSH): Glycoprotein of known composition; from anterior pituitary: Follicular cells of thyroid; stimulates release of thyronines.

Thyronines Thyroxine (T$_4$), Triiodothyronine (T$_3$): Iodinated derivatives of tyrosine (see figure 2.13); from thyroid: Most cells; increase metabolic rate, growth and development.

TRH: Thyrotropin Releasing Hormone—see Releasing Factors.

TSH: see Thyroid Stimulating Hormone.

Vasoactive Intestinal Peptide (VIP): Polypeptide (see figure 5.2); mainly from intestine but may be widespread (see table 1.1): Stimulates pancreatic bicarbonate secretion.

Vasopressin, Antidiuretic Hormone (ADH): Octapeptide (see figure 1.3); from hypothalamic neurosecretory cells: Water reabsorption in kidney.

Vasotocin (Arginine vasotocin): see Neurohypophysial Hormones.

VIP: see Vasoactive Intestinal Peptide.

CHAPTER ONE

COMMUNICATION AND CONTROL SYSTEMS IN ANIMALS

THE METAZOA HAVE OF NECESSITY DEVELOPED METHODS OF COMMUNICATION between their cells. In the early metazoa such communication systems enabled an organism to respond in a coordinated manner to stimuli from the external and internal environment. It can be assumed that this early form of communication involved chemicals which were already in the environment, either as by-products of the organisms' own activities, or of the activities of other organisms such as bacteria or plants. Such primitive mechanisms still persist, e.g. it is the accumulation of carbon dioxide which controls ventilation movements in insects and mammals. In all metazoa, however, the evolution of the nervous and endocrine systems has allowed the development of very sophisticated levels of coordination and integration.

1.1 What is endocrinology?
Endocrinology is that branch of physiology concerned with the study of hormones, the glands which produce them, and the target organs which respond to them. What then is a "hormone"? A classical definition might be: "Hormones are chemical substances produced by specialized ductless glands, and released into the blood where they are carried in the circulation to other parts of the body to produce specific regulatory effects". Recent studies have shown that some chemical substances appear to act rather like hormones but, for one reason or another, do not fit into the above definition. Perhaps, like some neurosecretions, they do not enter the general circulation (e.g. hypothalamic releasing factors), or do not enter

1

the blood at all (e.g. many invertebrate closed neurosecretory systems where the axons go directly to the target tissue), or, like prostaglandins (§2.2.5) for example, they are not necessarily products of specialized endocrine glands. Although it may eventually become necessary to re-define a hormone, we will here retain the classical definition given above but allow some flexibility in interpretation to cover such anomalies.

1.2   Nerves, hormones and neurohormones

The nervous system is ever present and always working; it is a discrete and localized system of rapid control, whereas the endocrine system often functions intermittently and exerts more diffuse and usually more pro-longed actions. The two systems are linked to ensure efficient regulation of the body. The simplest way to achieve this is by direct innervation of the endocrine cells by conventional nerves. This certainly occurs but is, in fact, the exception rather than the rule. Most endocrine cells receive no direct secreto-motor innervation, but are controlled at a distance by specialized nerve cells, called *neurosecretory cells*, or by other endocrine glands. All nerve cells are secretory in the sense that they elaborate and release chemical messengers at their synapses but, in conventional neurones, these transmitters are short-lived and need to travel only about 20 nm across the synaptic cleft. The chemical messengers released from neurosecretory cells, however, are often persistent and may act on much more distant receptors by entering the general circulation. A strict definition of a neurosecretory cell will not be given here. Indeed, in the light of recent findings it is very difficult to construct a precise definition which distinguishes clearly between endocrine and conventional neurones. Perhaps an adequate working definition is that a neurosecretory neurone is "a neurone which also possesses glandular activity".

In mammals, neurosecretory cells are restricted largely to the hypo-thalamus of the brain. In lower vertebrates and invertebrates, neuro-secretory cells are often more widely distributed throughout the nervous system (see below), but even in the higher invertebrates there is a tendency to concentrate the cells in the cerebral ganglia. Functionally, neuro-secretory cells occupy a dominant position in invertebrate endocrine systems and there are usually fewer peripheral (epithelial) endocrine glands than in vertebrates, and often none at all.

In many invertebrates the release of the neurohormones into the circulation involves little special structural organization but often neuro-secretory axons are found concentrated in particular sites, usually nerve tracts as in the molluscs, and in some cases, especially the arthropods, these concentrations of neurosecretory axons are elaborated into specialized structures analogous with the urophysis of teleost fish or the vertebrate posterior pituitary (neurohypophysis) where release occurs. These are often associated closely with the circulatory system and, if so, are

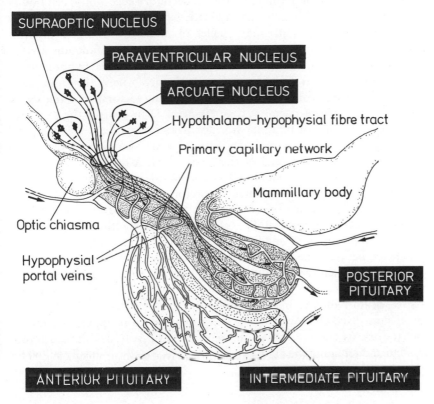

Figure 1.1 The anatomical relationship between the pituitary and the hypothalamus in a mammal. Neurosecretory cells in the paraventricular, supraoptic and arcuate nuclei of the hypothalamus send axons to the median eminence and the posterior pituitary, where they terminate adjacent to capillaries in these two structures. Neurosecretory hormones produced in the hypothalamus are released into the blood at these sites. The pituitary portal system consists of a primary network of capillaries in the median eminence, taking blood via the portal veins to a secondary network in the anterior pituitary. The hypothalamic hormones which control anterior pituitary function thus reach the anterior pituitary by the portal blood supply; the anterior pituitary has also a direct supply of blood (not shown in this diagram) from branches of the pituitary arteries. After Frye, B. E., in *Hormonal Control in Vertebrates*, Macmillan Press, 42, 1967.

termed neurohaemal organs. Examples in the arthropods are the insect corpora cardiaca (figure 6.1) and the crustacean sinus gland (figure 6.3), whilst in the annelids the infracerebral complex (§ 7.6.3) may also function partly as a neurohaemal organ.

The posterior pituitary of vertebrates (figure 1.1) is a complex neuro-haemal organ. It arises embryologically as a downgrowth of the forebrain, and contains the axon terminals of neurosecretory cells whose cell bodies lie in bilaterally paired groups (nuclei) within the hypothalamus; the supraoptic and paraventricular nuclei of amniotes, and the preoptic nucleus of fish and amphibia, produce peptides which function as true circulating hormones. Other neurosecretory cells in the hypothalamus have axon terminals in the median eminence where they discharge hormones (hypothalamic hormones or releasing factors) into the hypo-thalamo-hypophysial portal system (figure 1.1) to control the synthesis and release of anterior pituitary hormones. In many teleost fish, a second major neurosecretory system (the caudal spinal-urophysial system) is situated at the posterior end of the spinal cord. A distinct neurohaemal urophysis has only been identified in teleost fish but elasmobranchs also possess an elaborate caudal neurosecretory system. The physiological significance of this neurosecretory system remains, however, obscure.

What makes neurosecretory cells more suitable than conventional neurones for control of endocrine glands? One clue lies perhaps in the difference between the nature of nervous and endocrine (or neurocrine) control mentioned earlier. It is essential that all cells of a similar function within an endocrine gland act simultaneously to effect a sustained increased (or reduced) discharge of hormones. Nervous control, by virtue of its short-lived and localized nature, would therefore appear unsuitable, but the neurosecretory system, being intimately involved with the nervous system and retaining the ability to conduct electrically, is ideally suited for the purpose.

1.3 Hormone-like substances

1.3.1 *Neuronal peptides*
Peptides which appear to be very similar, if not identical, to known "true" hormones such as gastrin, cholecystokinin and vasoactive intestinal peptide, have been located by immunochemical techniques at widespread sites within the mammalian brain; similarly neurones which contain oxytocin, vasopressin, or one of the hypothalamic releasing factors, occur

Table 1.1 Some biologically active peptides found in mammalian brain.

Peptide Hormone	More usual or other locations
Oxytocin Vasopressin	Hypothalamus and posterior pituitary
Releasing Hormones (e.g. TRH, Gn-RH)	Hypothalamus
Substance P	Brain and gastrointestinal tract
Endorphins	—
Gastrin	Stomach
Cholecystokinin VIP (vasoactive intestinal peptide)	Gastrointestinal tract
Somatostatin	Hypothalamus, pancreatic islet and gastrointestinal D cells

outside the hypothalamus. Many other peptides are also found in the brain (table 1.1).

One important group of these peptides is known as the endorphins. The discovery of specific receptors for opiates such as morphine suggested that endogenous substances must exist which normally react (bind) with such receptors. Indeed, such endogenous substances, the endorphins (from *endo*genous and m*orphine*), have been isolated. The first of these to be discovered was named enkephalin and proved to be a pentapeptide of unusual structure. The amino acid sequence of enkephalin is contained within the pituitary polypeptide β-lipotropin. We shall return to this interesting point later (§ 2.2.2).

The physiological role of endorphins is still open to question but they may perhaps control feelings of pleasure or pain, or states of arousal or sleep. These and many of the other peptides found within the brain are unlikely to function as systemic chemical messengers but more likely as neurotransmitters, or modulators of neuronal function.

The ubiquitous nature of some peptides which have been regarded previously as specialized hormone molecules may have considerable significance in terms of the evolution of animal control systems. It is not possible to say whether the nervous system or the endocrine system arose first during the course of evolution and the fact that many neurones, widely distributed throughout the nervous system, have the ability to synthesize peptides does not help in deciding this question. This does suggest, however, that neurosecretory cells should not be regarded as unusual nerve cells in using peptides as chemical messengers. Indeed, perhaps this is a general or even primitive property of neurones? Furthermore there is evidence that the discharge of at least some neurosecretory cells is episodic, recalling the "all or none" characteristics of nerve transmission; it has been suggested that the regulation of the anterior pituitary might be related to the frequency, rather than the amplitude of releasing hormone secretion (see § 7.4.2).

1.3.2 Autocoids

A number of substances, known as autocoids or tissue factors, are known to act as "local hormones". They are synthesized, released and act locally on surrounding tissue; rapid degradation confines their area of influence. They are thus not carried into the blood circulation to distant sites as are true hormones. Perhaps the best known example of such an autocoid is histamine, but others are known, especially the kinins—a group of peptides including bradykinin. Bradykinin is formed in plasma and tissues by enzymic cleavage of a larger molecule (a zymogen?—see § 2.2.1) and is a potent vasodilator. It may play a role in normal inflammatory or allergic responses and may be responsible for the stimulation of pain fibres in injured tissue. This latter action may involve prostaglandins (§ 2.2.5) because aspirin, an inhibitor of prostaglandin synthesis, is an effective blocking agent. It has been proposed that these chemical messengers, which are quite widespread in occurrence, should be regarded as part of a so-called "paracrine" system in which products of cells act on immediate neighbours. Although this term has gained some acceptance it does not distinguish clearly between paracrine secretions and neurotransmitters.

1.3.3 Pheromones

We suggested at the beginning of this chapter that chemical communication is probably a very basic feature of metazoan life and, although we are concerned mainly with internally secreted messengers of the body, or hormones, we must mention the existence of other forms of chemical messengers which are secreted externally. Such messengers, or *pheromones*, are chemicals or groups of chemicals, which are secreted by one animal and affect the physiology and/or behaviour of another member of the same species. Another group of chemical messengers is called the *allomones* and they act in a similar way but this time the responding animal is reacting to chemicals produced either by a plant or an animal of another species. It is now realized increasingly that these forms of intraspecific and interspecific communication are important in the social behaviour and reproductive activity of many animals (mammals and insects provide many especially good examples). Pheromones and allomones are not in a strict sense part of endocrinology (perhaps exocrinology?), and space does not allow a detailed treatment of them here. Nevertheless, we should perhaps regard these informational molecules as closely akin to hormones and operating according to those principles governing all forms of chemical communication.

1.4 The study of endocrinology

The classical direct experimental approach to endocrinology involves the *ablation* (removal) of a suspected endocrine gland. This should result in a clearly defined complex of symptoms (a syndrome) which can be alleviated or reversed after subsequent *replacement* by re-implantation of the presumed endocrine gland, or by treatment with extracts of the gland or with the pure hormone. This particular approach is not always possible. It may be, for instance, that it is technically too difficult to remove the suspected endocrine cells; the surgical difficulties and/or trauma may be too great—the tissue may be too diffuse or embedded within other non-endocrine tissues. This is often true of neurosecretory cells unless they lie clustered within a superficial or otherwise accessible part of the nervous system.

More indirect methods involve histological and histochemical examination of suspected endocrine tissue using either the light or electron microscope. Such studies may be useful in suggesting the chemical nature of any secretion (§ 2.1) or in assessing the relative activity of cells (§ 3.1.2). In particular, it may be possible to correlate variations in the histological/ultrastructural or histochemical features of the cells with physiological processes or events in the animal. Data of this sort must, however, be interpreted with caution: such correlations do not prove endocrine activity, nor do they indicate the nature of any relationship between the putative hormone and the physiological process it is thought to control. A response evoked by a hormone must be studied in detail to determine whether it is a primary effect (a direct response of a target tissue to that hormone) or whether it is a subsequent or secondary effect consequent on an earlier event either in that target tissue or some other. For example, brain hormone (activation hormone) stimulates moulting in insects (a secondary effect) but its primary action is to cause ecdysone production in the prothoracic glands (§ 6.1.1). In living organisms (in contrast to controlled experiments *in vitro*) many hormones are present simultaneously; potential target tissues are rarely exposed to only one hormone but rather to a changing spectrum of them. Hormones may interact with each other so that one hormone may antagonize or potentiate the action of another. When two hormones act in concert to produce an effect they are said to be *synergists*; this may involve a balanced interaction such as in the synergism between ecdysone and juvenile hormone in controlling development in larval insects (§ 7.7.2). In this interaction the presence of one hormone alters qualitatively the target response to the other. Often the combined response of the target organ to two hormones acting together may be greater than the sum of the individual responses to the hormones—they are then said to be *potentiative synergists*. Indeed the combined action of two hormones may elicit a response which neither hormone can produce on its own. Thus, in mammals, growth hormone exerts a lipolytic action on adipose tissue only in the presence of adrenal glucocorticoids. Finally, the action of one hormone may "prime" a target organ to respond to a second hormone—even in the absence of the first hormone (see, for example, § 4.2.1 and 7.3). These interactions between hormones are usually dose-dependent; as is demonstrated most clearly in the hormonal control of insect metamorphosis, where the titre of juvenile hormone is the determining factor which regulates the direction and speed of development. Thus, when a hormone is studied either *in vivo* or *in vitro* the possibility of any one or more of these types of interactions occurring must be considered. Indeed, it is clear that one reason for the occasional failure of experiments to demonstrate a hormonal response *in vitro*, or to give the same result as is seen *in vivo*, could be the provision of an inadequate culture medium or the lack of necessary synergist(s).

Eventually, the detection of the hormone in the blood and its purification, characterization, and chemical synthesis are natural progressions in the study of endocrinology. It should be clear from this brief account that endocrinology demands a wide repertoire of skills—both manipulative and analytical.

1.4.1   *Comparative endocrinology*

Comparative endocrinology is akin to comparative physiology or comparative anatomy; it is a study of hormones and the tissues which produce and respond to them in different species of animals. Thus it serves to elucidate the evolutionary relationships between hormones themselves and between the species studied. This function of comparative endocrinology is of great value but is perhaps essentially academic. Nevertheless studies of the organization of one species often help in the understanding of other, different species. Indeed, much of our understanding of the endocrinology of man has been gained from studies in other animals and these have often led to findings of considerable clinical importance.

1.5 Hormones and evolution

The study of hormones and evolution is concerned with the evolution of endocrine glands, hormone molecules, carriers or precursors, target organ receptors and their responses. We shall deal with one example—the neurohypophysial hormones of vertebrates—partly because enough is known about their structure and distribution to generate reasonable (if necessarily tentative) speculation on their evolution.

The characteristic neurohypophysial hormones of mammals are vasopressin and oxytocin. These peptides are very similar molecules, differing in amino acids only at positions 3 and 8 (table 1.2). In fact, all the jawed vertebrates so far examined possess two neurohypophysial hormones which are quite similar to those of mammals: all are octapeptides, but amino acid substitutions are seen at positions 3, 4 and 8. Such close structural conformities suggest that these peptides might have evolved from a common ancestral form, which is probably represented by the single neurohypophysial hormone found in cyclostomes—arginine vaso-

Table 1.2 Amino acid sequence of the known neurohypophysial hormones.

Parent molecule	1 Cys	2 Tyr	3 ..	4 ..	5 Asn	6 Cys	7 Pro	8 ..	9 Gly	(NH$_2$)

Peptide	Amino acids in position		
	3	4	8
Basic (= Vasopressin-like) peptides			
Lysine vasopressin	Phe	Gln	Lys
Arginine vasopressin	Phe	Gln	Arg
Arginine vasotocin	Ile	Gln	Arg
Neutral (= Oxytocin-like) peptides			
Oxytocin	Ile	Gln	Leu
Mesotocin	Ile	Gln	Ile
Isotocin (= Ichthyotocin)	Ile	Ser	Ile
Glumitocin	Ile	Ser	Gln
Valitocin	Ile	Gln	Val
Aspartocin	Ile	Asn	Leu

After Heller, H. (1974) *Gen. Comp. Endocr.*, **22**, 315–332.

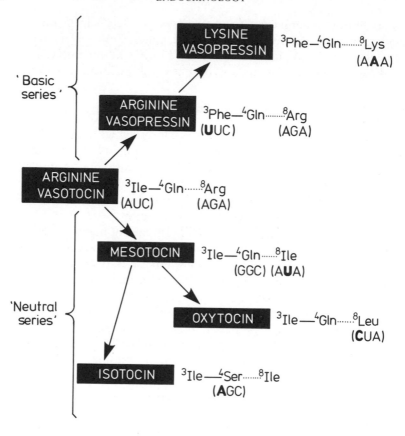

Figure 1.2 Molecular evolution of neurohypophysial hormones. The presumptive ancestral molecule, arginine vasotocin, could have given rise to the "basic" and "neutral" series of peptides by successive mutations affecting single bases of the genetic code. Possible changes in the mRNA codons are indicated in bold letters for the amino acid substitutions involved at each step. (Note that other combinations are possible in some cases, since some amino acids have several alternative codons.)

tocin. Reference to the mRNA code for the amino acids concerned lends support to this hypothesis (see figure 1.2): arginine vasopressin could have evolved from arginine vasotocin by a mutation affecting a single base in the mRNA codon for isoleucine (i.e. AUC to UUC); lysine vasopressin, the peptide of Suiformes (pig, peccary, hippopotamus) probably is the result of a more recent mutation in mammals. The origin of oxytocin and the other "neutral" peptides is less than clear, but a similar, albeit more

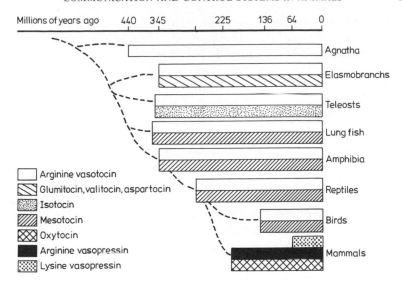

Figure 1.3   A phylogenetic tree of the main vertebrate groups showing the distribution of the neurohypophysial hormones. Note that this is a gross extrapolation of data available for a small number of species in each group. After Barrington, E. J. W., in *An Introduction to General and Comparative Endocrinology* (2nd edition) O.U.P., 104, Oxford, 1975.

tentative, scheme can be constructed (figure 1.2). The possible phylogenetic relationships of the vertebrate neurohypophysial hormones are shown in figure 1.3.

At the level of target organ evolution we can make the generalization that a hormone usually has more than one target tissue. This means that receptors for a hormone have therefore evolved in different tissues, which has led to diversification of hormone function. Perhaps it was easier to evolve new receptors in tissues than to develop new hormones? In any event, a study of comparative endocrinology suggests most strongly that it is the target organs which have changed most during evolution, not the hormones themselves. Indeed, it can be argued that there would be a strong selective pressure against changes in the molecular structure of hormones; amino acid substitutions are relatively infrequent in the "active" parts of hormone molecules compared with the biologically "inactive" parts or carrier components. Instead, the target organs have evolved to meet the requirements imposed by changes in the internal and external environment. For example, there is considerable evidence that in those land vertebrates which normally show drinking behaviour (dipsogenia), the brain contains (dipsogenic) receptors for angiotensin II (§ 8.2.1) which will react with injected (intraperitoneal) angiotensin to induce drinking behaviour. This response occurs in most reptiles, birds and mammals (but only in those which normally drink), but not at all in amphibia. It is argued therefore that these dipsogenic receptors for angiotensin appeared at a later stage in vertebrate evolution than the amphibia. Stenohaline fish do not possess dipsogenic receptors for angiotension either, but euryhaline fish, like the eel, do respond to the hormone by drinking. In these fish, however, the dipsogenic receptors occur in a different part of the brain from those in land vertebrates and must therefore have evolved quite separately. Thus receptors in the brain have evolved independently for the same peptide (in this case, angiotensin II) at least twice in the vertebrates as an adaptation to the external environment. We cannot be sure however whether drinking behaviour is elicited normally by circulating peptide acting on receptors outside the blood-brain barrier, or whether an endogenous brain renin-angiotensin system is involved.

1.6   The APUD concept

Professor A. G. E. Pearse of the University of London has suggested that all vertebrate peptide hormones (including neurosecretory hormones) are produced by a series of cells which have a common embryological origin and possess common cytological and ultrastructural characters. The cells are known by the acronym "APUD" which describes their most important and constant cytochemical properties—"Amine content and/or Amine Precursor Uptake and Decarboxylation". Other cytochemical and ultra-structural characteristics can be identified but will not be described here. However, the presence of cytoplasmic storage granules (100–350 nm in diameter) should be mentioned. Pearse lists over 30 cell types in the APUD series—some examples of these are given in table 1.3. He suggests that all these cells derive embryologically from neural crest or from neuroectodermal tissue. Indeed, there is good evidence for the migration of neural crest tissue to form the adrenal medulla and the C cells of the thyroid.

The synthesis and storage of amines is an important property of all APUD cells and forms the basis for one of the methods of identifying these cells; they fluoresce after freeze-drying and application of formaldehyde vapour. The association between this property and that of the synthesis

Table 1.3 Some of the endocrine cells thought to belong to the APUD series.

Cell location	Primary product(s)
Pituitary	ACTH
Pituitary	MSH
Pancreatic islet B (β)	Insulin
Pancreatic islet A (α_2)	Glucagon
Pancreatic islet D (α_1)	Gastrin, Somatostatin
Pancreas D_1	VIP
Thyroid and ultimobranchial C	Calcitonin
Stomach G	Gastrin
Stomach D	Somatostatin
Stomach EC	5-HT, Substance P
Duodenum S	Secretin
Duodenum K	GIP
Intestine EG	Enteroglucagon
Small intestine EC	5-HT, Motilin, Substance P
Intestine D	Somatostatin
Intestine I	CCK
Large intestine EC	5-HT
Carotid body type I	Dopamine
Adrenal A	Adrenalin
Adrenal NA	Noradrenalin

VIP, vasoactive intestinal peptide. CCK, cholecystokinin. GIP, glucose-dependant insulin-releasing peptide. 5-HT, 5-hydroxytryptamine.

After Pearse, A. G. E. (1976) in *Peptide Hormones* (J. A. Parsons, ed.) Macmillan Press.

and secretion of polypeptide hormones, however, cannot be explained on a molecular, biochemical or evolutionary basis.

The APUD concept is not unchallenged. It can be argued that as the neuroectodermal origin of all APUD cells (especially those in the intestine) has not been proved, the common features of these cells may be a consequence of convergence resulting from the evolution of similar function in cells of diverse origin. Some of the evidence concerning the relatedness of the chemical structures of peptide hormones in vertebrates, however, appears to support the APUD concept (§ 2.2.2). It is intriguing that cells which appear to have all the characteristics of APUD cells have been described in the intestine of a wide range of invertebrates but, as yet, their possible endocrine function has not been established clearly nor have their embryological origins been determined.

CHAPTER TWO

THE STRUCTURE AND FUNCTIONING
OF ENDOCRINE CELLS

2.1 The structure of endocrine cells

2.1.1 *Endocrine cells that produce proteins and peptides*
Endocrine cells which synthesize proteins and peptides are remarkably similar in their general structure throughout the animal kingdom, although the degree of development of particular cell organelles may differ depending on the amounts of protein synthesized.

A diagrammatic generalization of a typical protein- or peptide-producing endocrine cell is shown in figure 2.1. The major characteristics are the rough endoplasmic reticulum, a prominent Golgi complex and (usually) large numbers of storage droplets. The hormone synthesized on the ribosomes is segregated in the reticulum, transported through its lumen to the supranuclear region, concentrated, and formed into secretory granules in the Golgi complex. A detailed account of the synthesis of insulin in the β-cells of the pancreas is given in section §2.2.1.

An interestingly different example of an endocrine cell which produces a proteinaceous secretion is the follicle cell of the vertebrate thyroid gland. Thyroxine is not a protein, but it is synthesized as part of a large globular mucoprotein, thyroglobulin. This protein does not accumulate intracellularly but is discharged at the apical surface of the follicle cells (figure 2.2) and stored extracellularly (see §2.2.4). The general features of the cell conform to those outlined for other endocrine cells with proteinaceous secretions but, as might be expected, the structural characteristics associated with storage of the hormone in granules are absent.

2.1.2 *Endocrine cells that produce steroids*
The steroid-synthesizing cells of both invertebrates and vertebrates share a

14

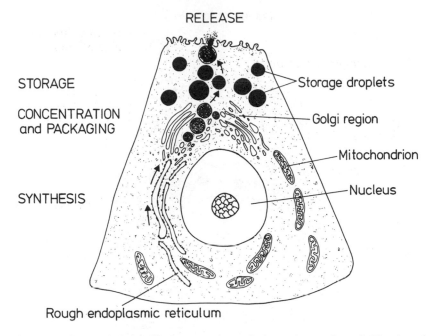

Figure 2.1 Diagram of the ultrastructure of a typical protein-secreting cell. The sites of synthesis, packaging and release are indicated. After Fawcett, D. W. *et al.*, (1969) *Rec. Prog. Horm. Res.*, **25**, 315–380.

characteristic fine structure which is quite different from those cells which produce proteins (figure 2.3). Typically, cells engaged in steroidogenesis have extensive smooth-surfaced endoplasmic reticulum; many of the dehydrogenations and hydroxylations involved in steroid biosynthetic pathways (figures 2.9; 2.10) take place here. The Golgi complex is often prominent. Steroid hormones, unlike peptides, are not usually stored prior to release; the cytoplasmic lipid droplets which are commonly seen in these cells contain precursor materials, such as cholesterol esters. The mitochondria, which are often variable in size, have an internal structure quite unlike those of other cells: the cristae have a tubular, or vesicular appearance reminiscent of smooth endoplasmic reticulum—and very different from the typical lamellar arrangement of "normal" mitochondria. This characteristic of steroidogenic mitochondria is related to their specialized function: in steroid hormone biosynthesis, several hydroxylation reactions take place within these organelles. Interestingly,

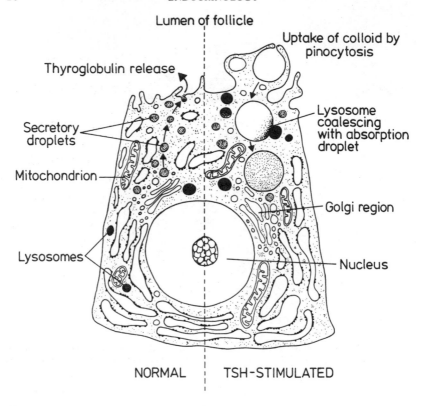

Lumen of follicle

Uptake of colloid by
pinocytosis

Thyroglobulin release

Secretory
droplets

Lysosome
coalescing
with absorption
droplet

Mitochondrion

Golgi region

Lysosomes

Nucleus

NORMAL   TSH-STIMULATED

Figure 2.2 Diagram of the ultrastructure of a thyroid epithelial cell in the normal (left) and TSH-stimulated (right) states. After Fawcett, D. W. *et al.*, (1969) *Rec. Prog. Horm. Res.*, **25**, 315–380.

when this activity ceases—for example in adrenocortical cells after surgical removal of the pituitary (hypophysectomy)—the mitochondrial morphology gradually changes to that seen in non-steroidogenic tissues.

2.1.3 *Neurosecretory cells*
Neurosecretory cells may be regarded as neurones with glandular activity (§ 1.1). As such they possess features in common with conventional neurones, including a similar morphology and an ability to conduct electrically. Neurosecretory cells which innervate their target organs directly have more or less conventional synaptic endings (e.g. the neurosecretory neurones which release the plasticization hormone in *Rhodnius*:

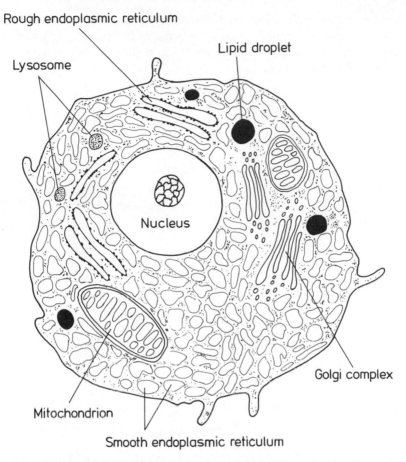

Figure 2.3 Diagram of the ultrastructure of a steroid-secreting cell. After *Research in Reproduction*, **3**, No. 5., International Planned Parenthood Association.

§8.1.2), but most release their secretions into the blood. These secretions are stored in characteristic membrane-bound granules, usually 100–300 nm in diameter.

There are basically two types of neurosecretory cells. *Peptidergic* cells synthesize and release peptides such as oxytocin or adipokinetic hormone and possess storage granules of around 300 nm in diameter (or larger); hypothalamic neurones producing releasing hormones have smaller granules (around 100 nm in diameter). In the second category are neurosecretory cells which are called *aminergic* because they secrete biologically active amines such as adrenalin, 5-hydroxytryptamine and dopamine. These amines are also stored in membrane-bound vesicles, of around 100 nm in diameter.

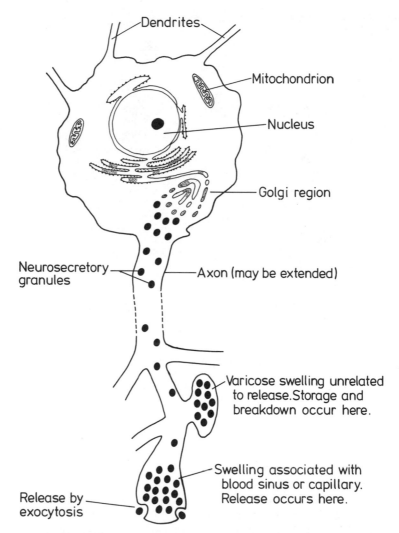

Figure 2.4 Simplified diagram of a neurosecretory cell. Neurosecretory material is synthesized in the cell body (perikaryon) and transported along the axon to terminal swellings where it is released into the circulatory system. Not drawn to scale.

The secretory granules of neurosecretory cells are elaborated in the Golgi complex after synthesis of the hormones at the membranes of the rough endoplasmic reticulum. In this matter, neurosecretory cells resemble other protein-producing cells; they usually possess a well defined Golgi complex, abundant rough endoplasmic reticulum and, of course, numerous membrane-bound vesicles (figure 2.4). In mammals and arthropods the axons running from the perykarya are often varicose at intervals and vesicles are found in abundance in their dilations (see figure 2.4). The material stored in these non-terminal dilations is not immediately lost to the pool of releasable hormone but freshly synthesized vesicles in the main axon and terminal dilations appear to be released preferentially. The non-terminal dilations are thought to represent both sites of vesicle storage, until such time as a massive release of hormone may be required, and sites of vesicle degradation. The mechanism by which stored neurosecretory granules can be recognized as being "too old" and fit only for destruction is unknown.

2.2 Hormone synthesis

2.2.1 *Protein and peptide hormones*

Many peptides or protein hormones are synthesized as larger molecules which subsequently undergo limited proteolysis to yield the smaller, active

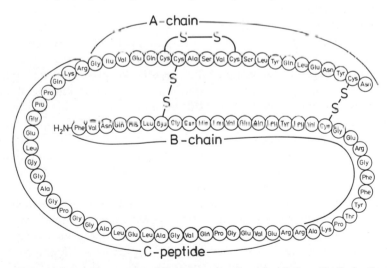

Figure 2.5 Amino acid sequence of bovine proinsulin. After Steiner, D. F., in *Peptide Hormones* (J. A. Parsons, ed.) Macmillan Press, 49–64, 1976.

hormone. The parent molecule, or prohormone, may be a polymer of the active hormone or it may form a basis for attaching various sub-units of protein hormones in the correct configuration (see figure 2.5). Prohormones often have little or no biological activity compared with the actual hormone and thus are analogous to intestinal proteases (zymogens) which are also synthesized and released as inactive precursors; the prohormone angiotensinogen, for example, is actually released as an inactive molecule (§8.2.1).

This type of peptide hormone synthesis is well illustrated in the production of insulin in the β-cells of the Islets of Langerhans of the pancreas. A precursor proinsulin molecule is synthesized in the endoplasmic reticulum and then cleaved enzymatically to form proinsulin. The molecule is folded, and disulphide bridges (–S–S–) are formed by sulphydryl oxidation between pairs of cysteine residues. Completed proinsulin molecules are then transferred to the Golgi region where packaging into granules and proteolytic conversion to insulin and C-peptide begins (figure 2.6). Many other peptide hormones are synthesized initially as large molecules; these include gastrin, glucagon, oxytocin and vasopressin, and the lipotropin/corticotropin family of peptides (see below). One important feature of the putative precursors (where their structure is known) is the presence of a pair, or more, of basic residues at the sites where cleavage is required to liberate the active molecule or hormone. The structure of proinsulin (figure 2.5) exemplifies this feature in that lysine and arginine residues separate the A-chain from the C-peptide and two arginine residues separate the C-peptide from the B-chain. The consistent occurrence of a pair of basic residues at cleavage sites in hormone precursor molecules suggests that intracellular trypsin-like proteases may play a special role in peptide hormone synthesis, but little is known of these enzymes or their control. Most peptide hormones are stored in membrane-bound granules. These granules are thought to facilitate transport within cells (especially neurones), offer chemical protection to the hormones, and may allow the more rapid release of large quantities of hormone than in those endocrine systems (e.g. steroidogenic tissues) where little hormone is stored and synthesis must precede release.

In vertebrates, neurohypophysial hormones are transported attached to carrier protein molecules called neurophysins; carrier proteins for other neurosecretory hormones may be widespread, but the evidence for their occurrence in invertebrate neurosecretory systems is circumstantial— although it is widely assumed that they exist.

The mechanisms by which the granules are rapidly transported in the

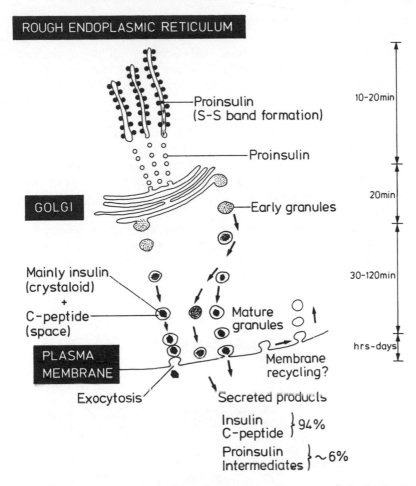

Figure 2.6   Schematic summary of the biosynthesis of insulin in pancreatic β-cells. The time scale on the right indicates the time required for each of the major stages in the biosynthesis. After Steiner, D. F., in *Peptide Hormones* (J. A. Parsons, ed.) Macmillan Press, 49–64, 1976.

cell (especially down long neurosecretory axons), or the mechanisms of release of the hormone from the granules into the blood, are not understood fully. One widely proposed (although not undisputed) mechanism of release is that of exocytosis whereby the granules approach the plasma membrane and the membranes of the granule and cell fuse to release the contents of the granule into the extracellular fluid (§ 2.3).

2.2.2 Families of peptide hormones

Close structural similarities between some hormones and groups of hormones have led to the idea that "families" of hormones can be identified in which the hormones of one family can be derived (in biosynthetic and/or evolutionary terms) from a single parent molecule; examples range from small groups such as glucagon/secretin (which, for example, in the pig share 15 amino acid residues at identical positions), cholecystokinin/gastrin (figure 2.7), and vasopressin/oxytocin (there is evidence that these are synthesized, each associated with their respective neurophysin carrier, from a single prohormone precursor), to the larger gonadotropin/thyrotropin and lipotropin/corticotropin families. We will discuss only the latter two examples.

The gonadotropin/thyrotropin family   The mammalian gonadotropins (LH and FSH) and thyrotropin (TSH) are each glycoproteins comprising two dissimilar glycoprotein subunits, α and β. In a given species the α subunits of LH, FSH and TSH have identical (or very similar) amino acid

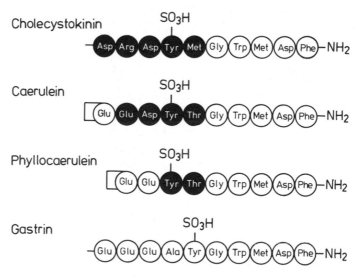

Figure 2.7. Amino acid sequence of porcine cholecystokinin and sulphated gastrin. The structures of caerulein and phyllocaerulein are shown for comparison. These latter two peptides can be extracted from frog skin and gastrointestinal tract and may represent the frog "gastrins". It is suggested that gastrin and cholecystokinin have evolved from a common caerulein-like ancestral molecule. Those residues differing from gastrin are shown by the dark circles. After Larson, L.-I. and Rehfeld, J. F. (1977) *Nature*, **269**, 335–338.

sequences. It is the β subunits which differ between the hormones and convey their specificity of action. Although the structures of the subunits differ, there are a sufficient number of similar amino acid sequences at identical positions in the molecules to support the concept that these glycoprotein hormones all derive from a common ancestral molecule.

The lipotropin/corticotropin family   At least seven of the pituitary peptides are considered to be members of the lipotropin/corticotropin family; β-lipotropin (β-LPH), γ-lipotropin (γ-LPH), adrenocorticotropin (ACTH), β-endorphin, corticotropin-like intermediate lobe peptide (CLIP), and α- and β-melanocyte stimulating hormone (α- and β-MSH). The general structures of these peptides are indicated in figure 2.8.

Although these peptides often display species variations in structure, within any single species they show sufficient similarities to suggest that they all derive from a common glycoprotein precursor, pro-opiocortin, of about 30 000 molecular weight. Recently, the nucleotide sequence of mRNA coded for bovine pro-opiocortin has been determined and it is possible to predict from this the amino acid sequence of pro-opiocortin itself. In general, this prediction is in good agreement with the known amino acid sequence of the peptides in this family. Pro-opiocortin appears to be composed of four repetitive units based on the MSH/ACTH core sequence (figure 2.8) which are separated by paired basic residues (see

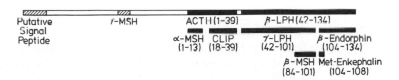

Figure 2.8 Schematic representation of the structure of bovine pro-opiocortin. The closed bars represent the regions for which the amino acid sequence is known, and the open and the shaded bars represent the regions for which the amino acid sequence has been predicted from the nucleotide sequence of the pro-opiocortin precursor mRNA. The locations of known component peptides are shown by closed bars: the amino acid numbers are given in parentheses. Adrenocorticotropin is a 39-amino acid peptide whose first 13 amino acids are identical in sequence with α-melanocyte-stimulating hormone (α-MSH) and whose 18–39 sequence is identical to corticotropin-like intermediate lobe peptide (CLIP). The α-MSH is acetylated at the NH_2-terminus and amidated at the CO_2H terminus. β-Lipotropin (β-LPH) is a 93-amino acid peptide whose first 60 amino acids are identical in sequence with γ-LPH and whose 61–91 sequence is identical to β-endorphin. The sequence 41–58 is identical to the 18-amino acid peptide β-MSH. The locations of γ-MSH and the putative signal peptide are indicated by shaded bars; the termini of these peptides are not definitive. After Nakanischi, S., et al., (1979) *Nature*, **278**, 423–427.

§2.2.1 above). An interesting finding here is the recognition in the predicted amino acid sequence of pro-opiocortin of a new MSH sequence (γ-MSH, figure 2.8); the physiological significance of this peptide remains to be determined.

The enzymatic cleavage of pro-opiocortin could release a large number of potentially active molecules. We know little of how such processes are controlled, or of the mechanisms by which unwanted products are broken down or inactivated. It is clear, however, that ontogenetic changes in the ratio of α-MSH, CLIP, β-MSH, ACTH and β-endorphin found in the mammalian pituitary do occur (although the changes in different species appear not to be always in the same direction). Thus, α-MSH and CLIP are the most predominant of these peptides in the human fetal pituitary, but almost disappear in the adult to be replaced by ACTH (this may represent an important qualitative difference in the control of adrenal function).

The existence of such families of peptide hormones is extremely important for our understanding of the way in which vertebrate peptide hormones have evolved. There is evidence of an increase in genome size during the early stages of chordate evolution, and in higher vertebrates this has resulted from duplication of genes, or groups of genes, rather than polyploidy. Thus, the structural gene for pro-opiocortin, for example, evolved probably by a series of gene duplications. Such a mechanism for peptide hormone evolution may have been a general feature in the vertebrates.

2.2.3   Steroids and insect juvenile hormones

There appears to be a common sequence of reactions which lead to the synthesis of vertebrate steroid hormones. Cholesterol, which is always the precursor molecule, is synthesized in the various steroidogenic endocrine tissues from acetyl CoA, via a pathway which involves mevalonate and squalene as intermediates. Steroidogenic tissues also obtain cholesterol directly, either from the blood plasma or by hydrolysis of cholesterol esters stored in cytoplasmic lipid droplets. Insects are unable to synthesize cholesterol, and therefore require a dietary supply of this steroid to synthesize ecdysone (see below). The pathways of steroidogenesis in vertebrate tissues are shown in figures 2.9 and 2.10. The conversion of cholesterol to pregnenolone and progesterone is common to all steroidogenic cells, but the further conversion of progesterone to andro-gens, oestrogens and adrenocortical hormones involves various oxidations, reductions and/or hydroxylations of the steroid. The enzymes

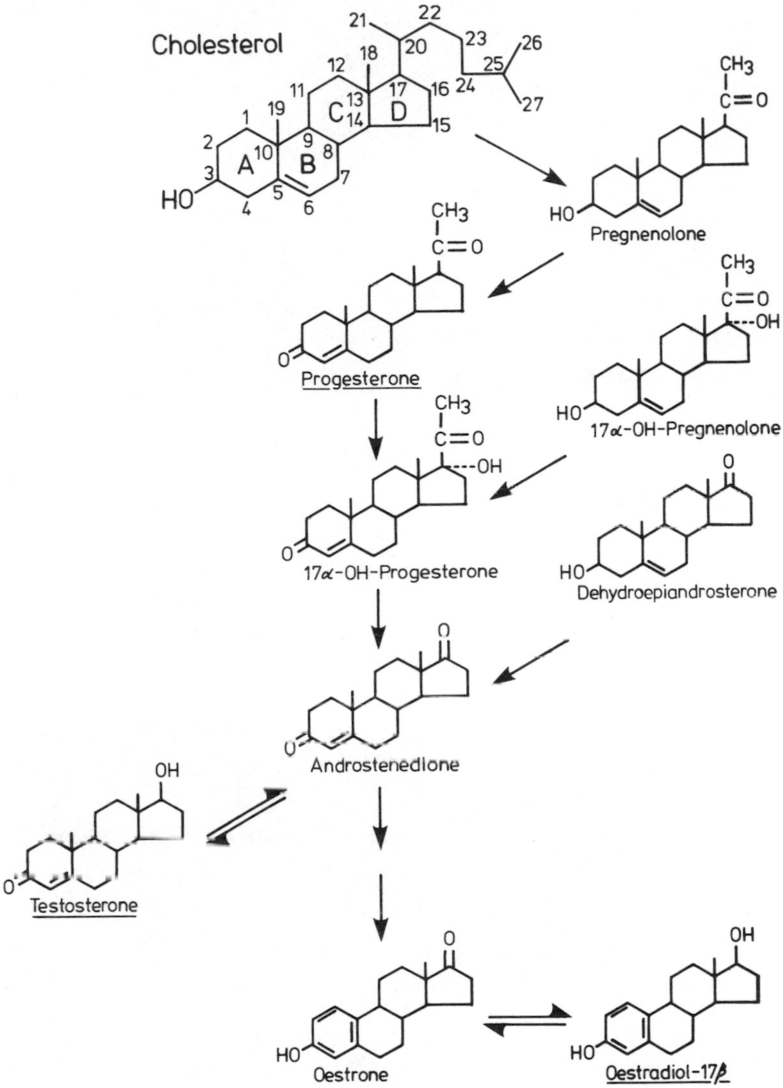

Figure 2.9 Pathways of biosynthesis of sex steroid hormones. The convention for designating the carbon atoms (numbers) and rings (letters) of the steroid nucleus and sidechain are shown on the cholesterol molecule.

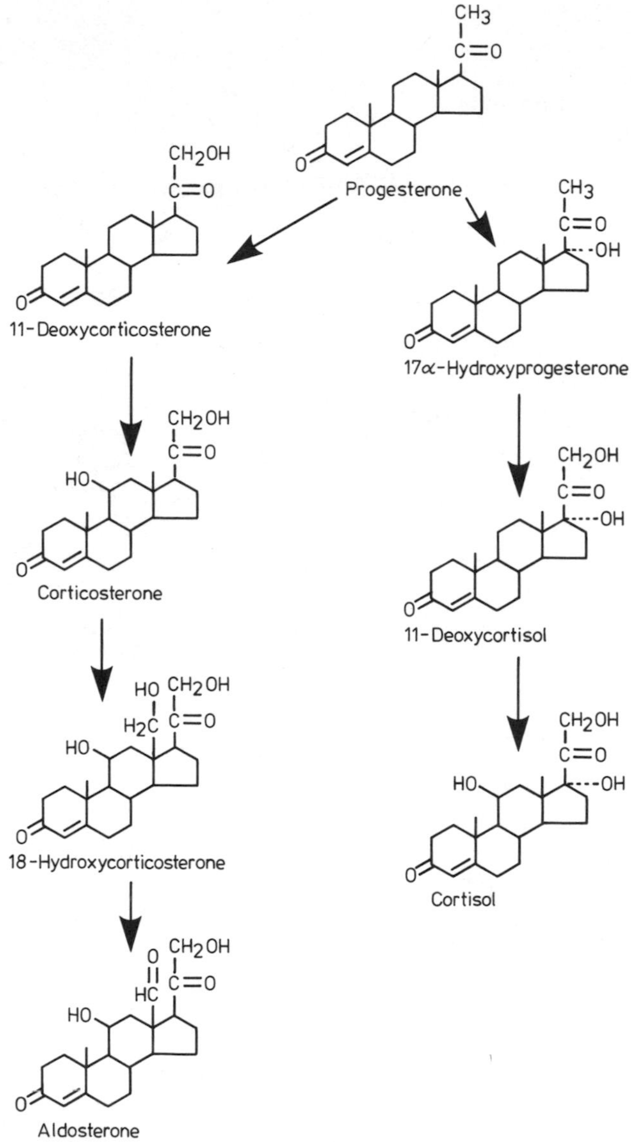

Figure 2.10 Biosynthesis of adrenocortical steroid hormones. The pathway from cholesterol to progesterone is not shown, but is identical to that given in figure 2.9. Adrenocortical cells also synthesize small amounts of androgenic and oestrogenic steroids, by routes similar to those shown in figure 2.9.

responsible for these metabolic conversions are distributed between the endoplasmic reticulum and mitochondria of steroidogenic cells. The presence or absence of particular enzymes determines the ability of different tissues and different species to synthesize particular steroid hormones. In man, some diseases are attributable to enzyme deficiency in such biosynthetic pathways: for example, congenital adrenal hyperplasia derives from a defect in the final stages of cortisol biosynthesis (figure 2.10). Cortisol normally controls ACTH secretion by a negative feedback (§ 2.3). The low level of cortisol secretion in such disease states leads therefore to compensatory increased secretion of ACTH which stimulates both growth (hyperplasia) and steroidogenic activity in adrenocortical tissue. The "block" in the biosynthetic pathway allows large amounts of steroid intermediates to accumulate, and these are metabolized to

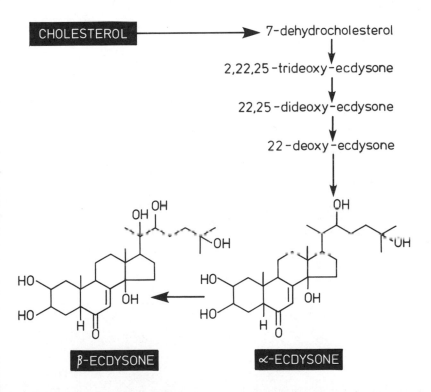

Figure 2.11 A tentative scheme for the biosynthesis of ecdysone. After Rees, H. H., in *Insect Biochemistry*, Chapman and Hall, 38, 1974.

androgens producing virilization; this is occasionally severe enough to cause a newborn girl to be mistaken for a male child.

The synthesis of steroids in invertebrates is not well understood. Although it is known that molluscs, echinoderms and arthropods can synthesize a wide range of steroids, only in the arthropods is there conclusive evidence that these steroids serve an endocrine function. The ovaries of insects and crustaceans appear to synthesize a variety of steroids

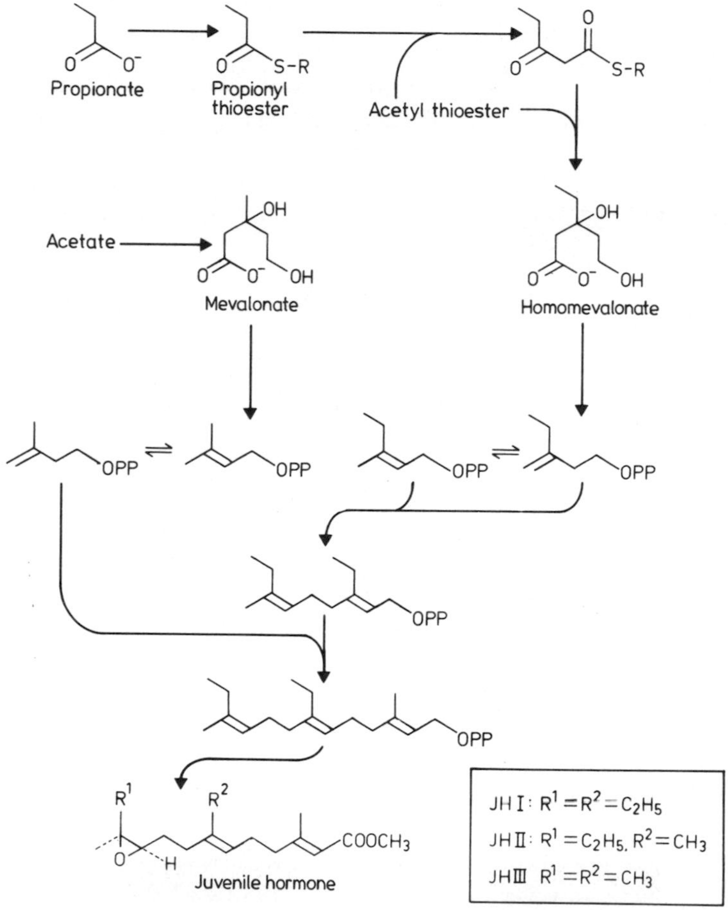

Figure 2.12 A tentative scheme for the biosynthesis of insect juvenile hormones. The scheme refers principally to the synthesis of JH I. After Schooley, D. A., *et al.*, in *The Juvenile Hormones* (L. I. Gilbert, ed.) Plenum Press, 101–117, N.Y., 1976.

which may all be intermediates in the synthesis of ecdysone. The classical example of steroid synthesis in arthropods is that of ecdysone in the prothoracic glands and Y-organ of insects and crustacea respectively. A tentative scheme for the biosynthesis of α- and β-ecdysone in insects is shown in figure 2.11.

The three known naturally occurring insect juvenile hormones are thought to be synthesized from acetyl or propionyl-CoA in the corpora allata. Although the complete biosynthetic pathway is uncertain, it is known that their skeletons are assembled from isoprenoid and homo-isoprenoid units. A tentative scheme for their synthesis is given in figure 2.12. Autoradiographic studies suggest that at least the final stages of juvenile hormone synthesis are undertaken by all the cells of the corpora allata and, although it is not possible to identify a specific site for the synthetic processes involved, the evidence suggests that they take place in the cytoplasm.

2.2.4 Tyrosine-based hormones

Thyronines The thyroid gland has the ability to sequester inorganic iodide from the blood against a considerable concentration gradient and to oxidize it to iodine; a reaction catalyzed by peroxidase. The reactive iodine then replaces hydroxyl sidegroups on the tyrosine residues of a large protein, thyroglobulin, to form thyronines according to the pathways outlined in figure 2.13A. The thyronines formed are mainly thyroxine (T_4, or 3,5,3',5'-tetra-iodothyronine) and T_3 (3,5,3'-triiodothyronine) and are attached to thyroglobulin in the ratio of about 5:1 per molecule of the protein. One molecule of thyroglobulin (mol. wt. 6.6×10^5) contains up to 5–6 molecules of thyroxine. The iodination process is thought to be initiated intracellularly prior to secretion of the thyroglobulin into the follicular lumen, but it may be completed extracellularly at the periphery of the follicular colloid in close association with apical microvilli of the follicle cells.

Catecholamines In vertebrates, the catecholamines, adrenalin and nor-adrenalin, are formed in chromaffin tissues. Noradrenalin is, of course, primarily a chemical transmitter at sympathetic nerve endings and in the central nervous system. These hormones are synthesized from phenyl-alanine by the pathways shown in figure 2.13B. In chromaffin tissue of the adrenal gland, two cell populations exist, one producing adrenalin and the other noradrenalin. The synthesized catecholamines are associated with

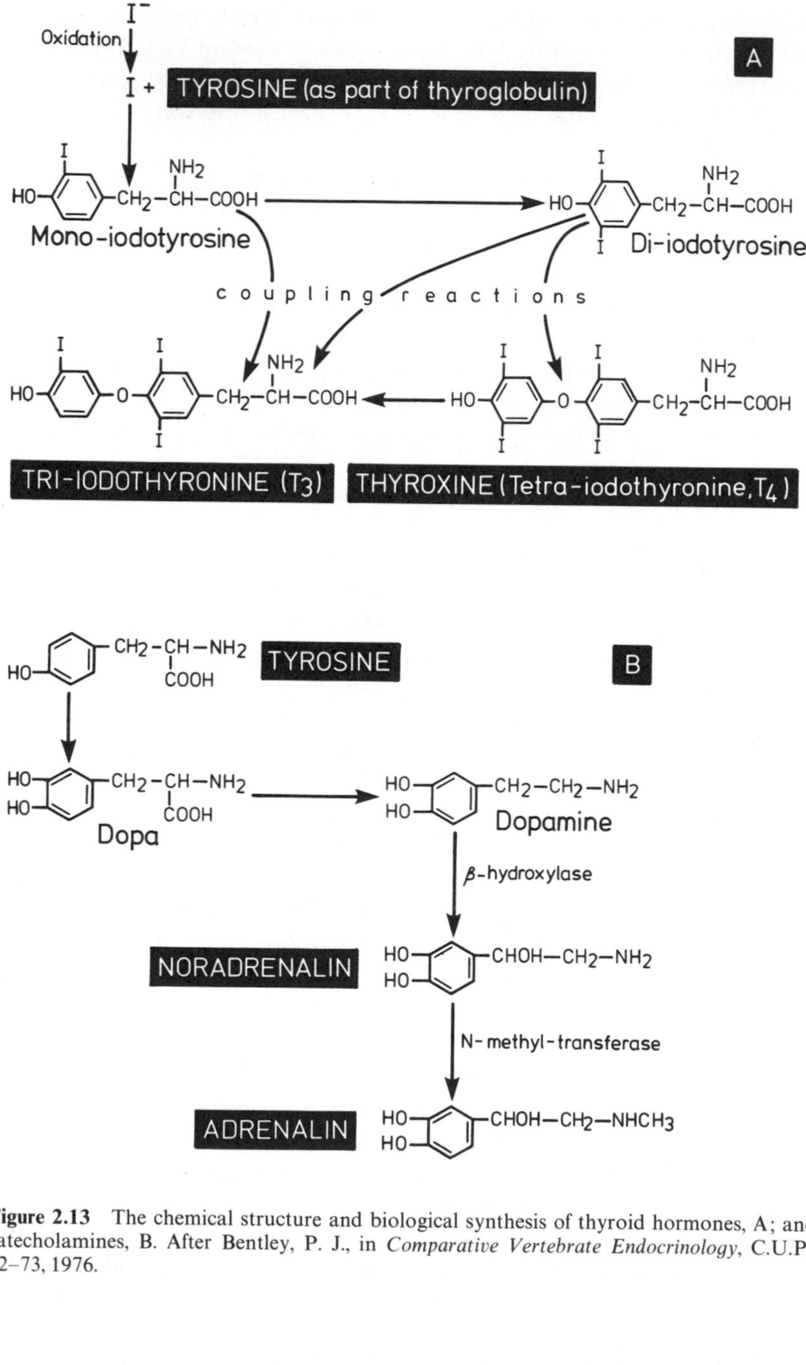

Figure 2.13 The chemical structure and biological synthesis of thyroid hormones, A; and catecholamines, B. After Bentley, P. J., in *Comparative Vertebrate Endocrinology*, C.U.P., 72–73, 1976.

ATP and a carrier protein (chromagranin) and are located in membrane-bound granules. Similar granules and storage complexes are found in adrenergic nerve endings and appear to be essential for the synthesis and storage of catecholamines. The production of dopamine (figure 2.13) occurs in the cytoplasm but its further metabolism occurs in the granules where the enzyme dopamine-β-hydroxylase is localized. In adrenal chromaffin tissue, the enzyme phenylethanolamine-N-methyltransferase is uniquely present to convert noradrenalin to adrenalin by methylation, S-adenyl methionine being the donor. The amount of this enzyme is controlled by corticosterone; hypophysectomy causes a marked decrease in activity whereas ACTH, or large doses of corticosteroid, restore activity. This enzyme is absent from adrenergic nerve endings and consequently it is only in the adrenal chromaffin tissue that appreciable quantities of adrenalin are produced.

Catecholamines and a wide range of bioamines are found in invertebrate endocrine systems but little is known of their synthesis, although it is generally assumed to follow pathways similar to those operating in vertebrates.

2.2.5 Synthesis of prostaglandins

Closely related unsaturated fatty acids, known as prostaglandins (PGs), are important components of many cellular processes. Originally, these substances were found in fresh human semen and attracted interest because they exhibited a wide range of physiological (and pharmacological) effects—from smooth muscle contraction, vasoconstriction, vasodilatation, and platelet aggregation, to the ability to mimic some hormones while blocking the effects of others. Prostaglandins are synthesized by most tissues of the body (figure 2.14). Their precise physiological role in many cases is not yet known, but within the last few years several important and independent functions have been identified: for example, they are involved in reproduction (ovulation, luteolysis, gamete transport, menstruation, abortion, parturition); control of body temperature by the hypothalamus involves PGs; the effects of several renally active hormones are mediated by prostaglandins produced within the kidney; prostaglandins play a role in blood clot formation, and in the inflammatory response. They may function as intracellular messengers, as local hormones, or as true systemic hormones. A number of anti-inflammatory, anti-pyretic (reducing fever) and analgesic drugs such as aspirin are thought to act by suppressing prostaglandin synthesis.

The prostaglandins are all 20-carbon fatty acids with a cyclopentane

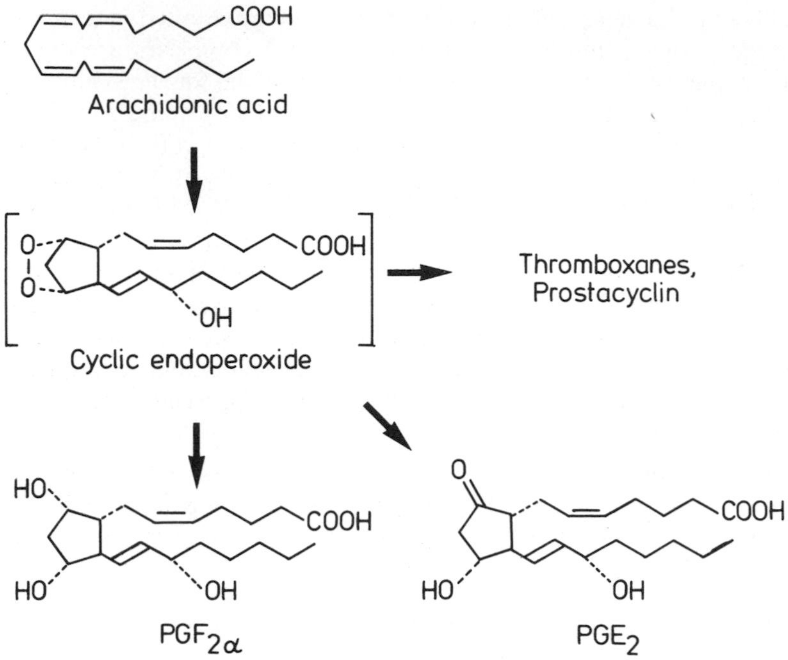

Figure 2.14 Biosynthesis of prostaglandins, thromboxanes and prostacyclin, from arachidonic acid.

ring, and are synthesized from essential fatty acids (e.g. arachidonic acid) by ring closure (figure 2.14). Synthesis occurs in the cytoplasm and the enzymes involved are microsomal. A large number of different prostaglandins are known and in fact two new classes of related biologically active lipids, the thromboxanes and prostacyclins, have been discovered very recently. These may prove to be of great physiological importance.

Although originally found in mammals, prostaglandins are known to be synthesized in many invertebrates and can be extracted in considerable quantities from some corals. Their physiological significance in invertebrates remains to be examined.

2.3 Release of hormones
The control of hormone secretion is complex and can involve nervous, endocrine and metabolic interactions. We have described already the need

for close integration of the nervous and endocrine systems in order to maintain a constant internal environment in the face of changing external conditions but, in general, we know less about the pathways by which external (exteroceptive) stimuli influence hormone release than we do about the mechanisms by which the internal (interoceptive) stimuli act. Of course, the interoceptive stimuli may often reflect external conditions, e.g. excess heat and/or desiccation will tend to increase the osmotic pressure of the blood.

Hormone release is usually triggered by precise or specific stimuli but, under conditions of "stress", non-specific stimuli of sufficient intensity and duration can cause hormone release and the endocrinologist must take this into account during experimentation. Further, release of hormones is often intermittent or cyclical (circadian, seasonal, annual, etc.), especially during reproductive development, and this has considerable practical significance in terms of measurement and interpretation of hormone titre; the timing and conditions under which the measurements are made are critical.

If hormones are to regulate the function of their target cells in a sensible manner, it is essential that the endocrine gland concerned should receive a constant supply of up-to-date information about the state of the target tissue. In fact, biological systems, at many levels of organization, respond in a manner which is determined not only by present and past stimuli but also by the response itself. In other words, they operate as closed loop systems; the release of hormone into the blood initiates in the target tissue some action which itself influences further release of hormone. Usually this feedback of information is negative in that it attenuates or stops further release (negative feedback) and this tends to bring the system towards a steady state. Such closed loop control mechanisms may be of various complexity; the concentration of the hormone in the blood (or some cellular product) may influence its own secretion—an ultra-short (direct) negative feedback loop (figure 2.15a); the hormone in the blood, or a metabolite under the control of the hormone, may influence a higher centre, the controller, in the CNS or another part of the endocrine system to modulate its own release directly—a short negative feedback loop (figure 2.15b); and finally, the target organ response may influence the release of hormone by acting at such a higher centre—a long negative feedback loop (figure 2.15c).

Little is known in detail of the controlling mechanisms for hormone release in invertebrates, but in vertebrates the controller is usually the hypothalamus which produces releasing or release-inhibiting factors to

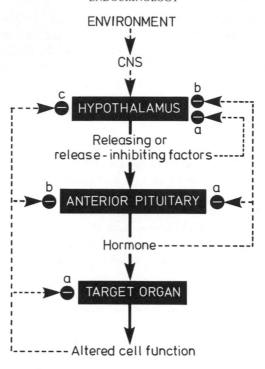

ENVIRONMENT

CNS

Figure 2.15 The control of hormone secretion in vertebrates by closed loop systems: *a*, ultra short negative feedback; *b*, short negative feedback; *c*, long negative feedback.

regulate the secretory activity of the anterior pituitary (figure 2.15). Positive feedback is known also, where the change or effect elicited by a hormone so alters the rate of release of that hormone that the net effect is greater. This type of feedback rapidly becomes unstable or climactic. Whereas negative feedback often underlies the maintenance of some preferred steady state (homeostasis), positive feedback enables some discrete event to be achieved rapidly once initiated. Ovulation and parturition in mammals offer good examples of endocrine coordination which relies on positive feedback (§ 7.4; 7.5).

While it has been recognized for many years that endocrine function usually involves complex closed loop systems, at least at the supracellular level, few studies have attempted to identify possible intracellular feedback mechanisms underlying either hormone release (see below) or hormone action (§ 4). This is an area of endocrinological research which requires both more work and a more enlightened attitude in terms of appreciating the closed loop nature of control in biological systems.

2.3.1 Stimulus-secretion coupling

The nature of the signals which control the activity of endocrine glands can be varied. Changes in the chemical environment of the endocrine glands through nervous, endocrine or metabolic events are usually the determining factors, but some neurosecretory cells are thought to respond directly to light. The mechanisms by which the arrival of the stimulus at the plasma membrane initiates release of hormone have been studied in some detail and a number of basic features appear common to most systems studied. Nervous stimuli, and some other chemical and hormonal stimuli, cause depolarization of the plasma membrane which alters its permeability to ions. In particular, the rate of Ca^{++} influx increases, and intracellular Ca^{++} pools may also be mobilized, so that the concentration of Ca^{++} in the cytosol rises markedly. In the adrenal medulla and the neurohypophysis, where hormones are stored in granules, the Ca^{++} stimulates movement of hormone granules towards, and their fusion with, the plasma membrane.

Modifications of this basic mechanism abound in different endocrine glands; for example, cyclic $3'5'$-adenosine monophosphate (cAMP) may be involved. Insulin will, again, provide a useful specific example. The mechanisms by which secretion is linked to the presence of those stimuli which effect release (stimulus-secretion coupling) are indicated in figure 2.16. Insulin release from the pancreatic β-cells is stimulated by glucose, GIP and glucagon, and inhibited by catecholamines. There are specific receptors (§4.1.2) on the plasma membrane for glucose (glucoreceptor) and for glucagon (and presumably for GIP). Glucose appears to cause membrane depolarization and influx of extracellular Ca^{++}. The consequent increase in intracellular Ca^{++} leads to granule movement and increased insulin release by exocytosis. This action of glucose is independent of cAMP. Glucagon, however, acts via an increase in adenylate cyclase activity; the increased levels of this cyclic nucleotide cause release of Ca^{++} from intracellular reservoirs, probably in the mitochondria. Precisely how an increase in intracellular concentration of Ca^{++} initiates release of insulin is unknown but, by analogy with the role of calcium in muscle, it is possible that Ca^{++} promotes the movement of granules towards the plasma membrane by stimulating the contraction of the microfilament-microtubular complex. Recently, however, it has been shown that insulin granules isolated from β-cells can be incubated with

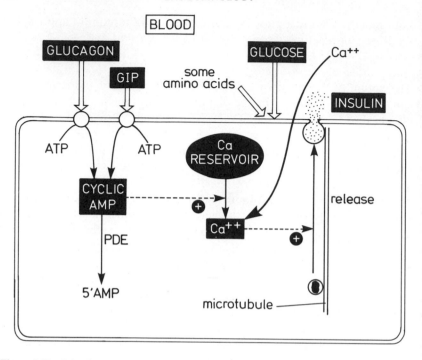

Figure 2.16 Stimulus-secretion coupling in pancreatic β-cells. Insulin release by exocytosis is stimulated by calcium which enters the cells during the action of glucose. Glucagon, and presumably GIP, raise the level of cAMP in the cells causing the release of calcium from intracellular reservoirs and thus potentiate the action of glucose. After Berridge, M. J. (1975) *Advances in Cyclic Nucleotide Research*, **6**, 1–98.

ATP and a purified plasma membrane fraction, and will release insulin in response to added Ca^{++}. This provides good evidence that at least one of the roles of Ca^{++} in excitation-secretion coupling is to cause fusion of granule and plasma membranes and subsequent rupture to release granule contents.

The difference in mechanism of stimulus-secretion coupling between glucagon and glucose raises several important questions. First, as a general point, it is now recognized that several intracellular signals, or *second messengers* (the first messenger being the external signal) are found in cells (§4.1.1). This last statement may prove to be a gross understatement of the truth—although we know something of the roles of cyclic nucleotides (cAMP, cGMP) and Ca^{++} as second messengers, it is conceivable that many inorganic ions could function in this manner. Second, the nature of the interactions between second messengers is important. In the pancreatic β-cell, glucagon or cAMP alone (in the absence of extracellular glucose) will not cause hormone release. In fact, glucagon does not stimulate insulin release in the presence of 3.3 mM glucose but does in 16.5 mM glucose. At concentrations of glucose below a critical level, cAMP concentrations increase, but insulin release does not occur. It would seem that in this system, cAMP plays a permissive role in secretion by potentiating the effects of glucose. This may have two important consequences. During starvation, when levels of blood glucose may fall below the critical value, glucagon will not cause an inappropriate release of insulin; and in the fed animal, glucagon release from the α-cells may prime the neighbouring β-cells to respond to the predictable increase in blood glucose by releasing insulin. This would represent a fine adjustment of the feedback mechanisms operating in the control of blood glucose levels (§ 5.2.3; figure 5.6).

There is much evidence to suggest that insulin release is also under considerable nervous influence via the splanchnic and vagus nerves. In particular, catecholamines inhibit insulin release and this appears to be related to a decrease in adenylate cyclase activity. Adrenalin, however, will also inhibit the glucose-stimulated release of insulin, but the mechanisms of these interactions are not understood fully.

The relative roles of cAMP and calcium vary considerably from tissue to tissue. For example the adrenal medulla, one of the earliest examples discovered of the dependence of secretory systems on Ca^{++}, operates rather like the pancreatic β-cell; acetylcholine released from the splanchnic nerve causes influx of extracellular Ca^{++} to initiate release of the granules which contain catecholamines. Cyclic AMP probably plays a minor role by releasing stores of intracellular Ca^{++}, increasing synthesis and, in the long term, by influencing cell hypertrophy and hyperplasia. On the other hand, in the anterior pituitary, although Ca^{++} influx (produced for example by K^+ depolarization) can cause hormone release without an increase in cAMP concentration, the major physiological control of hormone release probably occurs by a stimulation (by the various hypothalamic releasing factors) of the adenylate (or guanylate) cyclase systems. Finally, in the adrenal cortex, ACTH initiates the synthesis and release of corticosterone by a primary effect on adenylate cyclase activity and a second messenger role for Ca^{++} is less certain. The mechanism by which steroid hormones are released from cells is not clear; the amounts stored are small anyway, and synthesis and release of steroid must be activated at the same time. We will return to this particular example later when we consider the mechanisms of hormone action (§ 4.1.9).

The release of thyroid hormones represents an interesting departure from the mechanisms described above, in that the hormone is stored extracellularly in the colloid of the follicles within the thyroid gland. Because the thyronines are still attached to the thyroglobulin, this must first be taken back into the thyroid cells endocytotically (a reverse of exocytosis), where proteolytic digestion releases both thyronines and iodotyrosines. The latter are enzymatically deiodinated and recycled, only the thyronines being released into the blood; iodotyrosines appear to be protected from such enzymic attack as long as they remain attached to thyroglobulin. Stimulation of thyroid hormone release by TSH appears to depend on an increase in cAMP concentration within the follicle cells but how this stimulates endocytosis and colloid proteolysis is unknown.

CHAPTER THREE

ENDOCRINE ACTIVITY

3.1 Assessing endocrine activity

One of the essential components of practical endocrinology is the determination of endocrine activity. Endocrinologists ask the question "Is the gland (cell, tissue) actively secreting hormone?" An answer to the question may come from direct measurement of hormone release into the blood (see below § 3.2) but this is only possible if an appropriate method is available and then, if more than one source of the hormone exists, it does not enable us to differentiate between different sites of secretion.

3.1.1 *Histological methods*

Histological examination of endocrine cells, coupled with appropriate histochemical analysis, is used widely in assessing endocrine activity. Another approach is to weigh the endocrine organs, or to measure their volume. Such procedures, especially when they show changes in the parameter under study (density of histological staining, or other cytological changes, weight or volume of the gland) which can be related to some physiological event, are equivocal measures of endocrine activity; we cannot be certain that when an endocrine gland increases in size, or contains more histologically stainable material, that it has become more active. In other words, do such changes necessarily represent an increased synthetic and release capability? Is the hormonal product merely being stored and not released; which would be, of course, a decrease in endocrine activity in the accepted sense? This form of static analysis is inappropriate to dynamic systems. For example, in a single frame from a cine film we may recognize that a person is in a stance which is characteristic of walking, but we cannot be sure of the direction of movement, nor that the

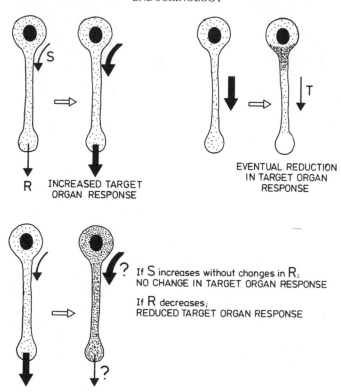

Figure 3.1   Simplified scheme for explaining possible changes (or lack of change) in amounts and distribution of cellular products in a hypothetical neurosecretory cell, in terms of rates of synthesis (S), transport (T) and release (R). Any permutation is possible. The thickness of the solid arrows indicates the magnitude of the rates.

motion would still be occurring in the next frame. A histological picture has similar limitations; it represents one moment fixed in time and cannot give us a true impression of dynamic events. A cell may double both its secretory and synthetic activity and we would expect to see no change in the amount of the stainable product within the cytoplasm. Similarly, if the amount of stainable material in the cytoplasm were to double, we could not be sure whether the rate of synthesis had increased, or whether the rate of release had decreased (see figure 3.1). In cells where material needs to be transported over considerable distances, then rates of transport become important too (figure 3.1). This is especially so for some neurosecretory cells.

One histological approach which attempts to overcome these criticisms is that of autoradiography. For example, accumulation of radioactive iodine by the thyroid, or of radioactively labelled cysteine by neurosecretory cells, can be used as a measure of endocrine activity, but such studies must be designed carefully and take fully into account the dynamic nature of the processes they seek to study—otherwise they become subject to the same criticisms as before. Thus, if it were desired to study the endocrine activity of a group of cells which synthesized a hormone containing cysteine, then the uptake of ^{3}H-labelled amino acid could be studied autoradiographically. If in one situation the number of cells showing ^{3}H-uptake within 2 h of the injection was double that in another, it would be uncertain whether this "increased uptake" was due to increased synthesis or decreased release (see figure 3.1). If however the *rate* of uptake of the label was measured this would give a rough index of endocrine activity but, alas, the true rate of uptake would be difficult to measure autoradiographically if the rates of transport and/or secretion were very rapid since freshly synthesized material would not be allowed to accumulate. Indeed it is necessary to study all three events. In practice this is best done by applying the radioactive label as a short "pulse", which can then be followed through the various processes of synthesis, transport and release from the endocrine system. These studies are time-consuming, often remain open to argument concerning their interpretation, and are applicable with certainty only to those systems where the chemical nature of the secretory material is known.

3.1.2 *Ultrastructural studies*
Quantitative electron microscopy is an attempt to assess the activity of cells by quantifying such features as the number of active Golgi zones, or the number of exocytotic vesicles (§2.2.1), as measures of synthetic or secretory activity. The results to date are promising but it is, again, time-consuming and laborious.

3.1.3 *Incubation methods*
Another method of assessing the activity of endocrine tissue is to incubate the tissue either in another animal, or in a suitable culture medium *in vitro*. The release of hormone from the transplanted tissue can be studied either as an observable effect *in vivo* in the host animal, or *in vitro* by co-culture of the endocrine tissue and its target, or by assay of the culture medium. Examples of some of these methods are given in figure 3.2 for the hormonal activity of the brain in nereid polychaetes (see also §7.6.3). The

in vitro approach has been used extensively in endocrinological studies of vertebrates and invertebrates, not only to study the release of hormones but also their synthetic pathways. One criticism of such experiments is that endocrine tissues probably behave differently *in vitro*, or when transplanted *in vivo*, from in the intact animal; not only because they are necessarily denervated and removed from their normal hormonal milieu but also because it may be difficult to reproduce *in vitro* certain critical conditions such as oxygenation, ionic environment and substrate supply (see also § 1.4).

3.2 Hormone assay

Historically, hormones were recognized as such by the characteristic biological activity they elicited. It may be that the biological activity observed is not the most important, or primary, action of the hormone, and clearly it is important to recognize that a single hormone may have a number of functions. Thus, it may act differently on different target cells, or on the same target at different concentrations, or act differently at different times (§ 3.3).

The concentration of hormone in the blood can be measured by one of two distinct forms of analysis; either measuring the actual number of hormone molecules present (an analytical approach which was not available to early endocrinologists) or by measuring the magnitude of the biological effect produced by the hormone. This latter method of assay, the biological assay or *bioassay*, measures the amount of hormone "activity" present in the sample irrespective of the number of molecules of hormone present.

3.2.1 *Bioassays*

For hormones of uncertain nature, or which are not available in pure form, the bioassay and its variants are an essential tool. This is often the case for recently discovered hormones, or those from lesser known species. Bioassay encompasses a wide spectrum of procedures, ranging from those carried out largely *in vivo* to those which utilize *in vitro* methods. An example of the former is the administration of LH to rats, which produces a graded increase in weight of the ventral prostate gland, measurable *post mortem*; a bioassay carried out entirely *in vitro* is described below (§ 3.2.5).

There are several disadvantages sometimes associated with bioassays. If the procedure relies on generating a response *in vivo*, the necessary maintenance of test animals is costly, labour intensive and time con-

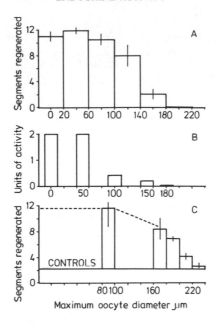

Figure 3.2 The assay of brain hormone activity in polychaetes by incubational methods. The brain of nereid polychaetes produces a single hormone which promotes regeneration of missing segments and inhibits sexual maturation. Regeneration of posterior segments decreases during gametogenesis (A) and this is viewed as an indication of reduced cerebral endocrine activity. This interpretation is supported by the observations that brains from donor females vary in their ability to inhibit gametogenesis *in vitro* (B) when implanted into isolated parapodia (organ culture), and also in their capacity to promote regeneration (C) when maintained *in vivo* in decerebrate worms which have had their posterior segments amputated. After Golding, D. W. and Olive, P. J. W., in *Comparative Endocrinology* (P. J. Gaillard and H. H. Boer, eds.) Elsevier/North Holland Biomedical Press, 118, 1978.

suming; in addition, such assays often show poor precision because of the inevitable variation in response between test animals (even those of the same inbred strain). Many of these problems can be reduced, and sensitivity also improved, by the use of suitable preparations of target tissue for short-term responses *in vitro* or, occasionally, for organ-culture studies (see figure 3.2).

3.2.2 *The use of radioactively labelled hormones for assay*
Great advances in science often only become possible when some new technique is developed. Radioimmunoassay is an outstanding example of this. Within the last fifteen years it has transformed much of endo-

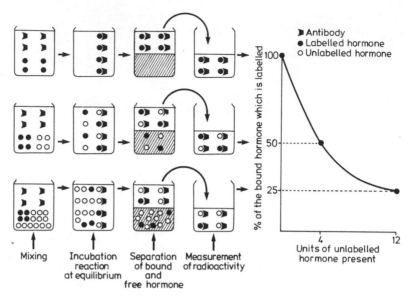

Figure 3.3 Simplified scheme for the radioimmunoassay of a hormone and the construction of a standard curve. Free and protein-bound hormone are separated (in this example) by the addition of charcoal, and centrifugation. The supernatant, which contains only protein-bound hormone, is decanted and its radioactivity measured: as the initial content of unlabelled (= nonradioactive) hormone in the original incubation is increased, the amount of labelled hormone in this supernatant will decline.

crinology, allowing direct measurement of hormone titres often several orders of magnitude lower than was possible using previous methods. Nor has its impact been confined to basic research: the ease of this technique, its low cost, and its facility for automation and the handling of large numbers of samples has led to its routine adoption in clinical situations. Medicine, and indeed the biological sciences generally, have benefited greatly from the advent of the radioimmunoassay—a debt that was acknowledged by the awarding of the Nobel Prize for Medicine to Professor Rosalyn S. Yalow in 1977.

Radioimmunoassays depend for their success on the extreme sensitivity of radiochemical methods; their great reproducibility and precision derive from the simple chemical stoichiometry on which they are based. Radio-actively-labelled and unlabelled (to be measured) hormones are allowed to compete for a limited number of binding sites, either on a specific antibody against the hormone (radioimmunoassay, RIA) or on a naturally occurring specific binding protein for the hormone (competitive protein binding assay, CPBA) (see figure 3.3). The reaction must take place in the presence of an excess of hormone, so that at equilibrium the ratio of bound radioactively labelled hormone to bound unlabelled hormone equals the ratio of the initial concentrations of the labelled and non-labelled hormone. After the addition of dextran-coated charcoal, the smaller, free molecules of hormone are adsorbed, and can be separated by centrifugation from the supernatant, which contains only hormone bound to antibody. The radioactivity of the supernatant is thus a measure of the proportion of labelled hormone which is bound; it will decrease as the initial concentration of unlabelled hormone increases. By then constructing a standard curve as in figure 3.3, the hormone content of an unknown sample could be assessed by measuring the ratio of the radioactivity in the bound phase to the total radioactivity (the % bound, as in figure 3.3) and making reference to the standard curve. (In practice, data are usually analysed by computer, and a linear function is derived in place of the exponential relationship shown in figure 3.3).

It would appear from the above account that the requirements for the development of a RIA for any hormone would be threefold: the hormone should be immunogenic, it should be available in pure form, and it should be possible to introduce a radiochemical label into the molecule. In fact, radioimmunoassays have been developed successfully for many molecules which are not themselves obviously immunogenic. The steroid hormones and cyclic nucleotides, for example, can be conjugated to high molecular weight carrier molecules (e.g. bovine serum albumin) and antisera raised against the conjugate. Antibodies are selected for their ability to bind the unconjugated steroid or nucleotide and thus allow its assay. In the CPBA the need for immunogenicity is of course not present, but the binding characteristics of the hormone to the protein must be as specific as possible. Usually naturally occurring proteins are used, for example those which exist in blood plasma for cortisol, or progesterone (see § 3.4.1); adrenocortical tissue can be used to prepare a specific binding protein for cyclic AMP. In general, the specificity of binding is not as high as that with antibodies, and samples often need to be purified before analysis. Both methods of assay require a radioactively labelled form of the hormone, which must be indistinguishable from the natural (unlabelled) hormone in terms of its binding characteristics. The radioisotope of choice for peptide and protein hormones is ^{125}I since it can be introduced by substitution into their tyrosyl residues with relative ease and high specific activity. Methods for the assay of non-protein hormones, such as steroids, originally used either radioactively labelled antibodies (the measurement now is of free and bound antibody), or tritiated (^{3}H-) forms of these hormones; more recently, iodinated (^{125}I) tyrosine methyl esters of such compounds have been employed because the specific activities attainable are greater, and their radioactivity can be measured more cheaply and conveniently than that of tritium labelled compounds.

3.2.3 *Problems concerning the use of radioimmunoassays*

Radioimmunoassays are now available for many hormones and other compounds of biological importance. Recently they have been used to measure juvenile hormone and ecdysone in insects and clearly, as more invertebrate hormones are characterized, the use of RIA in the study of invertebrate endocrinology will increase.

In most vertebrate studies, the results of RIAs agree well with conventional bioassay data. In some situations, however, gross discrepancies appear between these two methods of analysis. Two examples will suffice to illustrate the general problems: in experiments designed to investigate the half life of hormones such as ACTH and PTH, conventional bioassay data often gave times which were much shorter than when RIA was used for the measurements. It appeared that the RIA measured biologically inactive "ACTH" and "PTH" and thus gave an inaccurate estimate of the half life of the *active* hormone. For example, the biological activity of the PTH molecule depends only on the first 34 amino acids (of the 84 in total). It is known, however, that in human plasma the biologically inert chain of amino acid 35 to 84 is relatively long-lived compared with the authentic hormone. Moreover, oxidation of methionine residues in the molecule destroys the biological activity but the immunopotency may be unaltered. Second, it was shown that the use of RIA to measure the titre of growth hormone (GH) in blood from a wide range of vertebrates, including humans, was often invalid: biologically active GH in blood plasma was present in vastly greater amounts than the detectable immunoreactive GH. It may be that the circulating form of the hormone is not fully reactive with the antisera prepared against the form of GH as it exists in the anterior pituitary (although GH stimulates the liver to produce somatomedins, it is not these factors which are responsible for the above discrepancies). The lessons to be learned from such pitfalls are clear. The introduction of any RIA (especially for peptides) requires initial validation by comparison with established bioassay techniques. Often discrepancies can be avoided if the antisera used are those raised against biologically active fragments of the hormone; for example, antisera raised against the β-chain of LH show virtually no "cross-reactivity" with FSH.

3.2.4 Radioreceptor assays

Recently, assays which share many of the virtues of RIA, while eliminating their major (potential) disadvantage, have been developed for several peptide hormones. In these assays a preparation of specific hormone receptor, derived from an appropriate target tissue, is used in place of the antiserum of the RIA. Receptors will only bind "biologically active" hormone: indeed that interaction is the basis of the hormone effect (see § 4.1.2). The receptor preparation is usually a crude plasma membrane fraction, isolated after homogenization and sub-cellular fractionation of a target tissue; for example LH can be assayed using corpus luteum membrane preparations.

3.2.5 Cytochemical bioassays

A number of highly sensitive cytochemical bioassays have been developed recently. These depend on specialized histochemical analysis of the actual target cells for the hormone, and can often be 2 or 3 orders of magnitude more sensitive than RIA. One reason for this increased sensitivity is that cytochemical assays are performed on small pieces of tissue, or even on thin sections of tissue, which therefore require lesser amounts of hormone. Precision is improved compared with conventional bioassays because assays are performed only on the target cells and the results are not made more variable, therefore, by the presence of non-responsive (non-target) cells. Because such small amounts of tissue are required, one animal provides sufficient material for the assays to be *within*-animal, and the variability of hormone response that exists *between* animals is removed.

The first successful cytochemical assays were based on the depletion of ascorbic acid either from the adrenal or the ovary in response to ACTH and LH respectively. Other cytochemical assays have been developed for TSH, CRF and PTH. That for TSH is quite simple. When TSH initiates endocytosis in the follicular cells of the thyroid, primary lysosomes are activated to fuse with the colloid-containing droplets to form secondary lysosomes. A chromogenic substrate (leucine 2-naphthylamide) for an intralysosomal enzyme (naphthylamidase) is included in the incubation medium. When the lysosomal membranes become more permeable under the action of TSH, more substrate reaches the lysosomal enzyme and more is hydrolyzed. The degree of colour development provides a measure of the amount of hormone. The accurate measurement of colour development (the absorbance change) requires that the tissue sections are of uniform thickness. A special cytospectrophotometer, which is rather like a spectrophotometer built around a microscope, is used to measure the absorbance.

Cytochemical assays are extremely sensitive but they are time-consuming and technically very demanding. Their general acceptance seems unlikely since they cannot compete with the "off-the-shelf" nature of modern RIA or CPBS but their use in specialists' hands, as a check on the validity of these analytical assays, or in assaying titres which are too low for such methods, may prove invaluable.

3.3 Dose-response relationships

The patterns of response to hormones may change dramatically with the titre or amount of hormone (the dose). This is a function of the interaction of hormones with receptors in their target cells (§4.1.2 and 4.2.1). When hormones have a number of different actions, the dose-response curves for each of these may lie far apart; therefore different actions will be evoked according to the concentration of hormone in the blood. For example, four important metabolic effects of insulin have almost completely

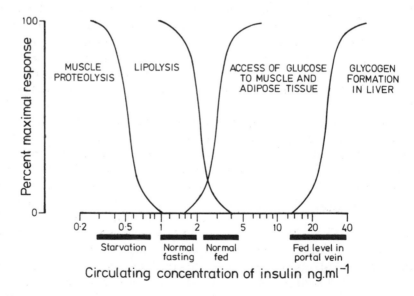

Figure 3.4 Estimated log dose-response curves of four important metabolic effects of insulin. After Parsons, J. A., in *Peptide Hormones* (J. A. Parsons, ed.) The Macmillan Press, 67–82, 1976.

separate dose-response curves (figure 3.4). It is clearly important that we know something of the normal levels of insulin under different conditions, so that we may discriminate between likely physiological effects, and those which are *pharmacological* (require hormone titres beyond the physiological range). The hepatic portal concentration of insulin in normal fasted humans is about $3\,\text{ng}\,\text{ml}^{-1}$ and the level in the peripheral circulation is about $0.5\,\text{ng}\,\text{ml}^{-1}$. The half-life of insulin is about 13 min, which interestingly does not differ between normal and diabetic individuals (see §5.2.5), with the liver and the kidney being the main sites of inactivation; about one half of the insulin reaching the liver via the portal vein is destroyed and never reaches the general circulation. The broad ranges of insulin levels under different conditions are indicated in figure 3.4 and it is clear that relatively small changes in titre can have striking metabolic effects. The diverse actions of insulin become more meaningful when one understands the dose-response relationships shown in figure 3.4.

3.3.1 *Variations in the response of the target tissue*

The response of a target tissue to a given concentration of a hormone, as described above, may be subject to considerable control by other factors, such as the stage of somatic and/or sexual development and differentiation, the time of day (or month or year), and the previous endocrine experience (see §4.2.1 below). For example, during metamorphosis in amphibia and insects, hormone sensitivity varies in a precise manner. In amphibia the early embryonic stages are insensitive to thyroxine, but towards the end of embryonic life sensitivity develops in such a way that the embryo can be thought of as a continually changing mosaic of thyroxine sensitivity; different tissues become responsive at different times but, as metamorphosis proceeds, some future adult tissues lose sensitivity. In the insects, epidermal cells are responsive to the morphogenetic action of juvenile hormone only in the larval stages—and even then, only for a short time at the beginning of each instar. In most adult female insects the fat body responds to juvenile hormone by synthesizing yolk protein but the fat body in larvae does not show this response. Clearly, during metamorphosis hormones may initiate responses in target cells but the in-built programme of each cell defines what the responses will be.

It is possible to postulate a number of mechanisms by which target response could be modulated. The presence or absence of receptors for particular hormones, or changes in the number of receptors, or the mechanism of second messenger action (§4.1.1) may all play a part. The rate of excretion or inactivation of the hormones may also be important (see below). Evidence for all of these possibilities will be presented in later sections of this book.

3.4   The fate of the hormone in the blood

The fate of a hormone once it has entered the blood is an important factor in determining its activity. The hormone may be taken up rapidly by its target organ (as we have mentioned for insulin), it may be activated or inactivated by enzymes present in the blood or other tissues, or it may be excreted. Initially, however, we must consider the form in which a hormone travels while circulating in the bloodstream.

3.4.1   *Binding proteins*

Many hormones are found in blood not as "free" molecules, but instead are "bound" to various proteins; this is especially true of steroid hormones, and also those of the thyroid. These so-called *carrier* proteins originally were thought to allow transport of hydrophobic steroids in the aqueous environment of plasma. Concentrations of different steroid hormones circulating in the blood vary, but in most cases are within the range 10^{-12} to 10^{-8} molar: although steroids might be regarded as being water-insoluble, extremely low concentrations such as these are easily attainable in aqueous solution by any steroid hormone, without the need for protein association complexes. Steroid carrying proteins (and those for other hormones) clearly have other primary functions, unrelated to "solubilization".

In general, the binding of hormones to blood proteins may be of two sorts: highly specific, high affinity binding to a protein present in relatively low concentration and therefore offering low overall capacity; or low-specificity, weak binding to commonly abundant proteins, such as albumens or lipoproteins, which offers a higher capacity. Examples of plasma proteins which show high affinity for different hormones include corticosteroid binding globulin (CBG) which binds corticosterone, cortisol, and less avidly, progesterone; sex-steroid binding globulin, which binds both testosterone and oestradiol; thyroxine binding globulin and insect juvenile hormone binding protein. Binding proteins create a buffer situation, where a large proportion of the hormone (often $>95\%$) is held in the bound form in equilibrium with a small "free" fraction. Only the free hormone can react with target cell receptors, or be metabolically degraded (often by the liver). As molecules of hormone leave this free pool, the displacement of the hormone-protein binding equilibrium ensures that a similar number of hormone molecules dissociate, so "topping-up" the free concentration.

The purpose of specific binding proteins is often claimed to be three-fold: to ensure that the hormone is transported in sufficient amount to activate the target organs; to protect the hormone from inactivation by enzymes present in the blood; and to add further specificity to the action of the hormone. In fact, the first two of these suggestions may be challenged. First, the solubility of insect juvenile hormones and all steroid hormones is high enough to not require this (see above). Second, the specific binding protein for insect juvenile hormone, while protecting it from non-specific hydrolysis of the methyl ester function, does not protect it from the specific esterases present in high activity in the blood at certain developmental stages. However, reduced rates of degradation of progesterone during pregnancy in some mammals are achieved by increasing the plasma concentration of a specific progesterone binding protein (see § 7.5.2). We might conclude that the main function of specific binding proteins (when they occur) is to add specificity to the action of the hormone by regulating the distribution of hormone between target issue and non-target tissue, or by affecting the relative distribution of hormones; hormone will only be released from one binding protein to another when the latter has a higher affinity for the hormone. For example, CBG allows aldosterone to react preferentially with target cell receptors because it binds corticosterone which is present in greater concentration than aldosterone. Thus those receptors in the target cells having a higher affinity for aldosterone than for corticosterone do not (inappropriately) attract corticosterone from CBG; the effect of aldosterone is therefore not obscured. Similarly in mammals, during pregnancy a plasma protein with high specificity for binding testosterone may afford protection to the mother from this steroid. In some insects the concentration of juvenile hormone binding protein varies during development and can be very high during periods when juvenile hormone titre is (and must be, from a developmental viewpoint) low. It is suggested in these cases that the binding protein may act as a scavenger to ensure that hormone titres are kept low, especially for particularly sensitive tissues.

3.4.2 *Peripheral activation of hormones*

A number of hormones are further modified in the blood or other tissues to form active or more highly active derivatives. Examples of such conversions include Angiotensin I to Angiotensin II (§ 8.2.1), thyroxine to triiodothyronine, testosterone to 5-α-dihydrotestosterone and other steroids (§ 7.2), and α-ecdysone to β-ecdysone (§ 6.1.1). Little is known of the factors which regulate the nature or rate of these conversions but they are important processes in the determination of hormonal activity.

3.4.3 *Inactivation or excretion of hormones*

In any system of chemical communication there must exist some mechanism for removing the chemical signal; it cannot be allowed to persist

1 day old, 5th instar larva

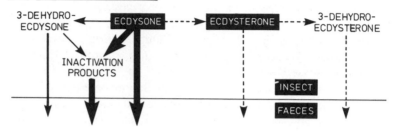

7 day old, 5th instar larva

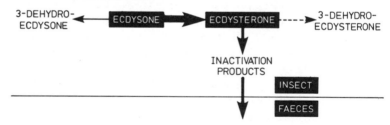

5 day old adult

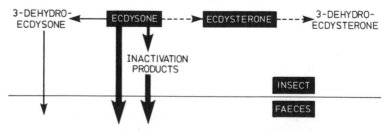

Figure 3.5 Pathways for the excretion and inactivation of ecdysone in the locust. The importance of the different pathways (indicated by the intensity of the arrows) varies with the stage of development. After Hoffmann, J. A., *et al.*, (1974) *Gen. comp. Endocr.*, **22**, 90–97.

indefinitely or a target organ would behave like a motor car with no brakes. In fact, the rates of removal of hormones from the blood are remarkably varied (from hormone to hormone, animal to animal in different physiological or developmental states, and from species to species). Hormones which influence developmental events generally tend to have longer half-lives than those which exert more rapid metabolic or physiological effects. Thus the half-life of adipokinetic hormone is about 30 min in the locust, or that of vasopressin is 15 min in the human (1 min in the rat); whereas thyroxine, for example, may have a half-life of around one week.

Hormones may be excreted from the blood into the urine either unchanged or as a derivative. For example, the vertebrate gonadotropins are excreted in a changed but still biologically active form in the urine whereas locust adipokinetic hormone is excreted rapidly by the Malpighian tubules but in an inactive form. Steroids may be excreted to some extent in an active unchanged form (figure 3.5) but like most hormones are subject also to degradation or inactivation in the blood or other tissues before they are excreted. Vertebrate steroid hormones, arthropod ecdysteroids, and to a lesser extent thyroid hormones (these are mostly de-iodinated), are converted largely to glucoside or sulphate esters but the relative importance of the different pathways may vary according to the stage of development (figure 3.5). Peptide and protein hormones are often subject to degradation by relatively specific proteases localized mainly in target tissues (and sometimes in blood); this latter point may be related directly to the problems of hormone action discussed in §4.1.10. The insect juvenile hormones can be inactivated by esterases in the blood (hydrolysis of the methyl ester function); the specific esterases, from which the hormones are not protected by the binding protein, show variations in activity during development and may, in some insects, provide a fine adjustment to the regulation of hormone titre. In other species, hydration of the epoxide function, which occurs in the tissues, may be more important in inactivating juvenile hormones.

CHAPTER FOUR

MECHANISMS OF HORMONE ACTION

NERVOUS COORDINATION CAN BE PRECISE: AN EFFERENT NERVE CAN stimulate a very discrete location by a direct route. Hormonal messages, in contrast, are broadcast widely, being carried in a medium which is essentially non-directional. In spite of this, endocrine coordination can also be directed precisely and need not affect large regions of the body. This capability is a function of target tissue; whilst blood-borne hormone molecules may be carried to (and even enter) most cells, the "message" is ignored in all except those equipped to receive it.

It is now recognized that hormones react with specific receptors associated with their target cells; the determination of target tissue specificity to a particular hormone is dependent upon the presence of such receptors. In general we can classify hormones into two categories, those which need to enter their target cells, and those which do not. This subdivision may not be as sharp as it seems—a point to which we shall return later (§ 4.1.10). Our main concern now is to determine how the interaction of the hormone with its receptor leads to an appropriate response of the target tissue.

4.1 Protein and peptide hormones

4.1.1 *Cyclic nucleotides and second messengers*

In 1958 Professor E. W. Sutherland and colleagues discovered an important intermediate which is involved in the mechanism of action of adrenalin. This compound, cyclic 3'5'AMP (cAMP), could elicit the hormone's glycogenolytic effect. It was established that adrenalin acti-

54

Table 4.1   Some hormones which are thought to act via cAMP.

Vertebrate hormones	Target	Invertebrate hormones	Target
Glucagon	Liver	Locust adipokinetic hormone (AKH)	Fat body and flight muscle
Adrenalin	Liver and muscle		
Vasopressin	Kidney	Arthropod hyperglycaemic hormones	Fat body/ hepatopancreas
Oxytocin	Uterine muscle and mammary gland	RPCH	Chromatophores
Parathyroid	Bone	Insect diuretic hormone	Malpighian tubules
Calcitonin	Bone	Bursicon	Haemocytes
ACTH	Adrenal cortex	Insect brain hormone	Prothoracic glands
LH	Ovary and testis		
FSH	Ovary and testis		
TSH	Thyroid		
MSH	Melanophores		
Hypothalamic releasing hormones	Adenohypophysis		

vated glycogen phosphorylase by first elevating the intracellular concentration of cAMP within the hepatic target cells; cAMP could be envisaged as the *second messenger*, responsible for the mediation of the intracellular actions of adrenalin (the "first messenger"). The significance of this research however, was to be much wider than this: cAMP was shown to be involved in the actions of a great many hormones (table 4.1). The elucidation of the second messenger concept proved to be a crucial watershed in endocrinology, and in recognition of this Sutherland was awarded the Nobel Prize for Medicine in 1971.

Cyclic AMP (figure 4.1) has been identified in bacteria as well as in all metazoa. It is formed from ATP in a reaction catalyzed by adenylate cyclase, and is degraded by hydrolysis of the 3'-ester function by a phosphodiesterase. Adenylate cyclase appears to be associated mainly with the cell membrane whereas the phosphodiesterase is distributed between the membrane and the cytosol.

Other cyclic nucleotides also are found in cells. Guanylate cyclase, which catalyses the formation of cyclic 3'5'-guanosine monophosphate

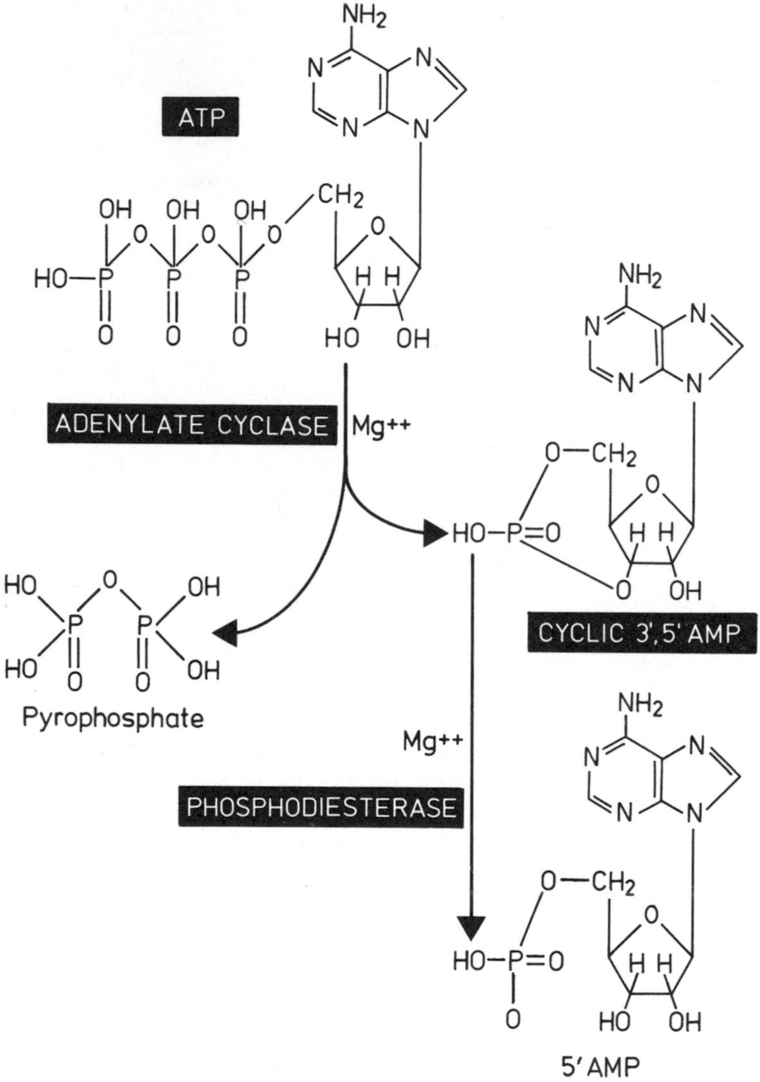

Figure 4.1 The formation and metabolism of cyclic AMP.

(cGMP) appears to be mostly in solution in the cytosol and the evidence of its direct activation by extracellular agents is less certain than for cAMP. It is conceivable, however, that guanylate cyclase is activated by intracellular messengers such as Ca^{++}. In general, there is little evidence of direct regulation of phosphodiesterases by hormones (but see § 4.1.9) but cGMP phosphodiesterase activity in photoreceptors is known to be activated by light.

4.1.2 *Receptors*

The effects of many peptide hormones, as well as the β-adrenergic responses to catecholamines, are mediated by stimulation of adenylate cyclase in the target cell. The hormone (an "agonist" in pharmacological parlance) binds reversibly to its receptor on the plasma membrane and forms a complex which is essential for its biological effect. If the receptor binding sites are occupied by another ligand which itself does not exhibit the biological action of the agonist (i.e. an "antagonist"), then the response to the hormone will either be blocked or will occur only if the hormone is present in a sufficiently high concentration to compete with the antagonist for the binding site. Demonstrable binding to the plasma membrane is of course not sufficient evidence that the binding sites are receptors with the potential for generation of second messengers. The binding characteristics must parallel the biological activity; the concentration of hormone required for half maximal binding should be in the normal physiological range of concentration of the circulating hormone; and antagonists of binding (whether competitive or non-competitive) should be antagonists of the biological response. In general, binding sites vary in their affinity for a hormone, and often two populations of such sites exist—a small number of high affinity sites and a larger number with low affinity for the hormone. The physiological significance of such an arrangement is not yet understood completely. Perhaps the low affinity binding sites represent non-specific binding and are not true receptors; their function may be to maintain a local high concentration of hormone close to the "true" receptors.

The specificity of hormone action depends on the distribution of receptors in the target tissues. Glucagon, for example, will stimulate glycogenolysis in liver but not in muscle; presumably muscle lacks the requisite glucagon receptor. The receptor and the adenylate cyclase response are linked in a complicated but largely unknown way. It seemed likely that they were separate distinct proteins—in tadpole erythrocytes, for example, adenylate cyclase activity is detectable before the sensitivity to adrenalin. However, adipose tissue ghosts (cells which have been lysed and retain the plasma membrane in the form of vesicles) respond to a variety of hormones (adrenalin, glucagon, LH, TSH and ACTH) by increased lipolysis (via an increase in cAMP) but the effects are not additive. This suggests most strongly that there must be separate receptors for all these hormones (could one receptor recognize such different molecules?) but these operate through a single adenylate cyclase system. Recently direct evidence has been obtained which clearly shows that β-adrenergic receptor and adenylate cyclase activity can be separated. N-ethylmaleimide was used to inactivate (irreversibly) adenylate cyclase of turkey erythrocytes, while leaving their β-receptors intact. The erythrocytes were then fused, with the aid of Sendai virus, to another type of cell which is known to have adenylate cyclase, but no β-receptors. The fused preparations showed β-receptor-dependent adenylate cyclase activity.

A number of models have been proposed to illustrate how hormone-receptor interaction affects adenylate cyclase activity. One of the most useful models is that which equates the mechanism with allosteric control of an enzyme which is composed of at least two subunits. The hormone represents an allosteric activator, the receptor a regulator subunit, and adenylate cyclase the catalytic subunit (figure 4.2). However, any theory of hormone-receptor-adenylate cyclase interaction must take into account the dynamic nature of the plasma membrane; the membrane should be viewed as a fluid mosaic containing globular proteins irregularly

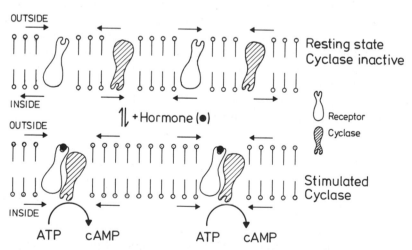

Figure 4.2 The mobile receptor hypothesis for the mechanism of adenylate cyclase activation by hormones. The receptors and the enzymes are viewed as separate entities which complex together only after the receptor is occupied by the hormone. After Cuatrecasas, P. (1974) *Ann. Rev. Biochem.*, **43**, 169–214.

embedded in a lipid matrix. Perhaps both receptor and enzyme (adenylate cyclase) molecules can each diffuse laterally within the plasma membrane, and occupancy of receptor sites by the hormone increases the affinity of the receptor for the enzyme (figure 4.2).

It should not be assumed that the interactions of peptide hormones with the receptors at the cell surface are understood completely. In particular, the chemical nature of receptors is not fully known, although their protein nature is suspected because proteolytic enzymes and peptidases destroy them. Several receptors are influenced by phospholipase: either they contain phospholipid, or binding to them is influenced by association with phospholipid in the membrane. Some receptors have carbohydrate moieties. Further, a number of quantitative aspects of receptor function are intriguing; for example, many hormones exert a maximum biological response by occupying only a small fraction of the receptor population. Such a phenomenon could mean that there are spare receptor sites but these should not be thought of as necessarily being inactive, since saturation of these sites with more hormone often leads to further increase in cAMP concentration. The presence of large numbers of receptors may well be an adaptation to ensure cell activation at low concentrations of hormone. However, in some tissues, hormone binding to the plasma membrane receptor and the biological response are correlated in such a way as to suggest that there are no spare receptors. Thus occupancy of receptors for angiotension II correlates with increased rates of aldosterone synthesis in the adrenal glomerulosa cell over the whole range of hormone binding. In some tissues the degree of receptor occupancy can lead to sequential biological responses. For example, the insulin-induced inhibition of lipolysis in fat cells occurs at very low receptor occupancy; stimulation of glucose metabolism is maximal when 2–3 % of the receptors are occupied; and stimulation of protein synthesis occurs at higher degrees of occupancy (see also figure 3.4).

Prolonged exposure of target tissues to high concentrations of some hormones (e.g. insulin, growth hormone, catecholamines and LH — § 7.3) is followed frequently by a decrease in the number of plasma membrane receptors. This effect is termed "down regulation" and may avoid over-response to the hormone; the mechanism is uncertain (but see § 4.1.10). A converse form of regulation, where an increase in hormone-specific receptors is stimulated either by the hormone itself or by another, is also known (§ 7.3).

Interestingly, the nucleotide GTP can influence the binding affinity of hormones for their receptors and, perhaps more importantly, can in many

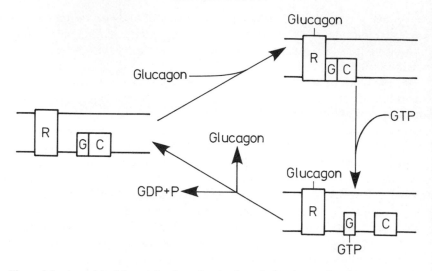

Figure 4.3 A model of the mechanism of activation of adenylate cyclase by glucagon and GTP. The glucagon receptor is represented by R, the catalytic unit of adenylate cyclase by C, and the GTP-binding regulatory unit by G. In the presence of glucagon the receptor (R) associates with the (GC) complex to form a ternary complex (RGC). In the presence of GTP, this complex dissociates to release the fully activated catalytic unit (C). From Martin, B. R., *et al.*, (1979) *Biochem. J.*, **184**, 253–260.

cases mimic the hormonal activation of adenylate cyclase (figure 4.3). Adenylate cyclase appears to have at least three sites at which individual ligands modify enzyme activity; the hormone receptor site, the catalytic site which reacts with ATP and Mg^{++}, and the nucleotide regulatory site. Nucleotide regulation of adenylate cyclase may represent a general feature of peptide hormone action but its significance is difficult to assess at present.

4.1.3   *Second messenger function of cAMP*

How does an increase in the intracellular concentration of cAMP bring about the diverse functions of all those hormones (table 4.1) which are thought to act by stimulating its production? Cyclic AMP is thought to act as a second messenger for the hormones by binding to an enzyme, protein kinase, and in doing so, activating it (figure 4.4). There are other possible actions of cAMP within cells—we have already mentioned its effects on Ca^{++} regulation (§ 2.3.1)—but most attention has been focussed on its activation of protein kinase. This enzyme, known as cAMP-

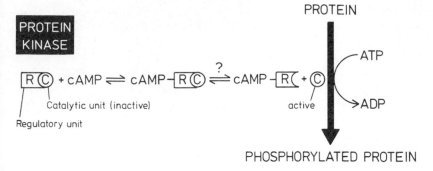

Figure 4.4 The activation of protein kinase (cAMP-PrK) by cyclic AMP. It is uncertain whether dissociation of the cAMP-enzyme complex is necessary *in vivo*.

dependent protein kinase (cAMP-PrK), is composed of a regulatory subunit (R), which binds cAMP, and a catalytic subunit (C), which contains the active site. The binding of cAMP to the regulatory unit *in vitro* causes dissociation of the R-C complex and the activation of the kinase, although it is not certain whether dissociation of the complex necessarily occurs *in vivo* (figure 4.4). A number of cellular proteins, and particularly enzymes, are known to undergo reversible phosphorylations but, of these, only a few are recognized as likely physiological substrates for cAMP-PrK (table 4.2) and rigorous analysis has proved such a role only for phosphorylase kinase. The importance of protein phosphorylation in the context of control theory is that it converts one form of the enzyme to another, which responds differently to changes in substrate (or allosteric effector) concentrations. In crude terms we talk of the enzymes being switched "on" or "off". This is inaccurate but is a convenient short-hand. The phosphorylation of phosphorylase kinase

Table 4.2 Some enzymes which are known to be subject to phosphorylation/dephosphorylation reactions.

1. Phosphorylase kinase (muscle)
2. Glycogen synthetase (muscle)
3. Triacylglycerol lipase (adipose tissue)
4. Pyruvate kinase (liver)
5. Cholesterol esterase (adrenal gland)
6. Phosphofructokinase (liver)
7. Pyruvate dehydrogenase (muscle)

Enzymes 1–5 are considered likely physiological candidates for cAMP-PrK.

(catalysed by cAMP-PrK) and its subsequent stimulation of glycogenolysis will be discussed in detail in the next section.

4.1.4   Glycogenolysis in muscle

The role of cAMP as a second messenger is best known in relation to the
effects of adrenalin on glycogenolysis in muscle. Here, the cAMP-PrK
phosphorylates a second protein kinase, phosphorylase b kinase. The
activation of this enzyme by cAMP-PrK is somewhat complex with two
distinct residues being phosphorylated (the regulation of enzyme activity
by phosphorylation at more than one site may prove to be a general
feature). Nevertheless, phosphorylase b kinase is activated by phosphorylation and catalyses the phosphorylation of glycogen phosphorylase
b to convert it from this inactive form to the active, "a" form (figure 4.5).

It is of interest to note that during electrical stimulation of muscle,
phosphorylase b kinase is activated by Ca^{++} in the absence of any
increase in the intracellular concentration of cAMP. Thus in skeletal
muscle, electrical activity (mediated via acetylcholine) brings about a
stimulation of glycogenolysis by an increase in intracellular concentration
of another second messenger (Ca^{++}); this also activates myosin ATP-ase
and consequently contraction. On the other hand, in smooth muscle the
relaxation effect of noradrenalin may involve cAMP but, in this case the
nucleotide-induced protein phosphorylation is thought to affect Ca^{++}-
transporting mechanisms and the intracellular concentration of Ca^{++}.

4.1.5   Glycogen synthesis

A second but related effect of adrenalin action on skeletal muscle is an
inhibition of glycogen synthesis. This too, is mediated by the increase in
cAMP within the muscle—in fact, by cAMP-PrK. The enzyme glycogen
synthetase exists in two forms which are interconvertible by phosphorylation and differ in their sensitivity to allosteric effectors such as
glucose-6-phosphate, ATP and inorganic phosphate. In resting muscle, the
"b" form (phosphorylated) is almost inactive but the "a" form (non-
phosphorylated) is almost fully active. The conversion of glycogen
synthetase a to b ("inactivation") is catalysed directly by the same cAMP-
PrK which we have already discussed (figure 4.5). Conversely, the
activation of glycogen synthetase ($b \rightarrow a$) is catalysed by a protein
phosphatase but, more importantly, by the same phosphatase which
dephosphorylates (and, in these cases, inactivates) phosphorylase b kinase
and glycogen phosphorylase. Thus glycogen synthetase activity is
switched off at the same time as glycogenolysis is initiated, and vice versa.

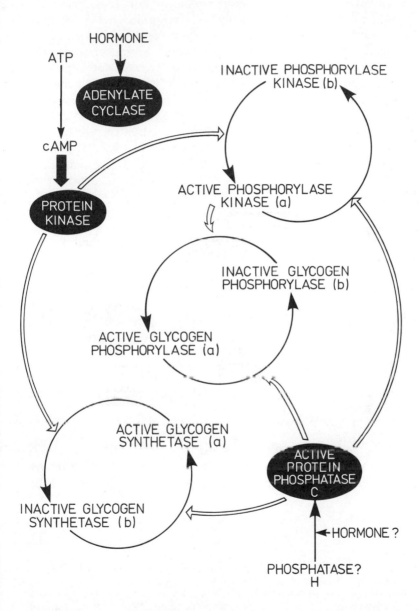

Figure 4.5 Interrelationships between the protein kinases and protein phosphatases of glycogen metabolism.

The situation *in vivo* is almost certainly more complicated than the above account might suggest. In particular, it is important that we discover how the activity of protein phosphatase is controlled, for this is clearly part of the closed loop system which we expect to find. Protein phosphatase exists in two forms: a high molecular weight form, termed protein phosphatase H, and a lower molecular weight form, protein phosphatase C. It is proposed that protein phosphatase H is activated by the release of an inhibitory regulator subunit to produce phosphatase C. This concept has been included in figure 4.5 but should be treated only as speculation. The primary regulator of protein phosphatase activity has yet to be determined, but it is tempting to imagine that insulin is a likely candidate.

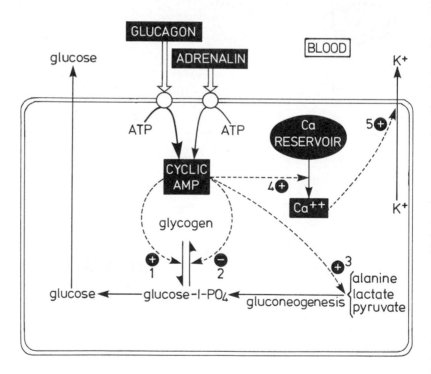

Figure 4.6 Interactions of cyclic AMP and calcium in the control of liver metabolism. Glucagon and adrenalin stimulate the synthesis of cAMP, which mediates the release of glucose by activating phosphorylase (1), by inhibiting the formation of glycogen (2), and by stimulating gluconeogenesis (3). Cyclic AMP may also stimulate the release of calcium from intracellular reservoirs (4) which, in turn, may stimulate the efflux of potassium (5). After Berridge, M. J. (1975) *Advances in Cyclic Nucleotide Research*, **6**, 1–98.

4.1.6 *Peptide hormones and the liver*

The liver represents a complex but nevertheless intriguing target organ for the endocrinologist to examine. It responds to many hormones and performs a central role in metabolism. It is important, therefore, that we consider how cAMP may act within it to control glycogenolysis, glycogen synthesis and gluconeogenesis.

Figure 4.6 represents a scheme for the second messenger function of cAMP in liver, based largely on analogy with muscle. Although the detailed actions of cAMP which have been elucidated in muscle are not as

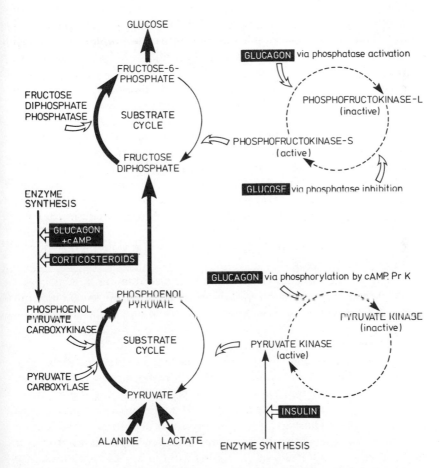

Figure 4.7 A tentative scheme for the hormonal control of gluconeogenesis in liver.

clearly established for the liver, it is generally assumed that the nature of the mechanisms operating is similar.

How glucagon stimulates gluconeogenesis is not fully understood but may involve cAMP and a cAMP-PrK (§ 4.1.3); two of the enzymes involved—phosphofructokinase and pyruvate kinase (figure 4.7)—show reversible phosphorylation.

Phosphofructokinase is an important regulatory enzyme in glycolysis (§ 5.2.1) and forms part of a substrate cycle with fructose diphosphate phosphatase (figure 4.7). The relative activities of these two enzymes determine the rate and direction of the overall flux. Thus increased gluconeogenesis could be brought about by an increase in activity of fructose diphosphate phosphatase or a decrease in that of phosphofructokinase. There is no convincing evidence that fructose diphosphate phosphatase is controlled by chemical modification of its structure but phosphofructokinase can be modified by phosphorylation-dephosphorylation reactions. In the liver of starved rats, most of the enzyme is in relatively inactive "*L*" form. When such rats are fed, the enzyme is found mainly in an active "*S*" form. The "*S*" form is derived from the phosphorylation of the "*L*" form. Phosphorylation is not cAMP-dependent, but livers from starved rats respond to perfusion with glucose by an increase in the "*S*" form. This response to glucose is decreased by glucagon but the mechanism is unclear. On the other hand, pyruvate kinase is also part of a substrate cycle (figure 4.7) and is another enzyme whose activity is regulated through reversible phosphorylation—but this time under the influence of cAMP. One effect of glucagon is to inactivate pyruvate kinase by phosphorylation and therefore shift the net flux in favour of gluconeogenesis.

Although some progress is being made in determining how glucagon stimulates hepatic gluconeogenesis, the exact mechanisms remain far from clear and the scheme presented in figure 4.7 should be considered tentative.

4.1.7   *Hormone interaction—glucagon and insulin*

The foregoing discussion has perhaps no more than scratched the surface in explaining the cellular action of some peptide hormones. Indeed, when we consider insulin we realize that in comparison with most other hormones, we understand only a little of its action at the molecular level. Insulin stimulates glucose uptake and glycogen deposition in muscle (in the absence of adrenalin) and stimulates glycogen deposition in the liver (in the absence of adrenalin or glucagon) without any observable change in cAMP concentration. Insulin does, however, decrease the elevation of cAMP caused by prior exposure to glucagon. The mechanism by which insulin antagonizes the cAMP-mediated action of glucagon is not understood, nor has an intracellular second messenger for insulin been found. On the other hand the only action of insulin which seems to be completely independent of any possible cAMP involvement—the stimulation of glucose uptake into cells—is not understood any better.

4.1.8   Hormone interaction—prostaglandins and peptide hormones

Prostaglandins of the E and F series (§ 2.2.5) have been studied extensively in relation to adenylate cyclase activity in many tissues. Interest arose because prostaglandin E_1 (PGE_1) could block the effect of lipolytic hormones which act by raising the cAMP levels in adipose cells. This, together with the observations that indomethacin (an inhibitor of PG synthesis) potentiated the effects of lipolytic hormones and that adrenalin caused a release of PG-like activity, led to the concept that endogenous PGs could serve to reduce the cAMP-mediated responses in adipose (and other) tissues, as part of a closed-loop system of control. However, in most other tissues PGs increase the production of cAMP and mimic the actions of many peptide hormones; PGEs, for example, are luteotropic and thyrotropic. It thus seems unlikely that PGs have a general role as local negative modulators of hormonal stimuli, although they do have that function in adipose tissue.

Prostaglandins have also been proposed as essential mediators of hormone action. The concentration of some PGs in the thyroid rises after TSH stimulation, and this effect is blocked by indomethacin; a similar situation occurs in the corpus luteum, in response to LH. In neither case, however, is the tropic hormone action (i.e. release of thyroxine, or progesterone) inhibited by indomethacin: thus PGs cannot play an essential role in these actions of TSH or LH.

Ovulation is stimulated by LH, and in this case PGs are obligatory mediators of at least some of the hormone's actions. Follicular rupture, and ovum extrusion in response to LH are caused by a rise in PG concentration within the follicle; when this is prevented by indomethacin, ovulation does not occur.

To summarize, it is clear that PGs are involved with the actions of several hormones. No general hypothesis, however, can account for the nature of the interactions observed: they vary with different hormones and tissues. Indeed different PGs quite often have opposing actions. For example, PGEs have a luteotropic effect on the corpus luteum, whereas PGFs are luteolytic (§ 7.4.1).

4.1.9   *Possible roles for other second messengers*

It was mentioned earlier that cAMP could act by affecting the intracellular concentration of Ca^{++}, and calcium itself can have a second messenger function in its own right (§ 2.3.1). In metabolically very active tissues such as the liver and adipose tissue, it seems that cAMP is usually the primary second messenger for peptide hormones and the involvement of Ca^{++} is

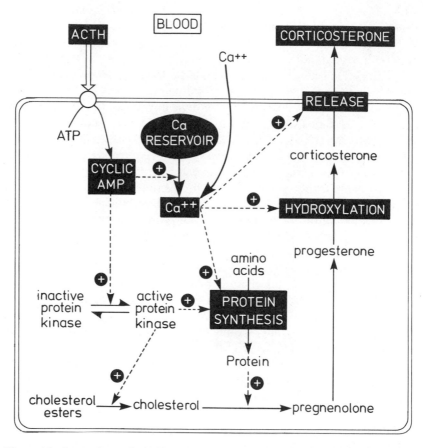

Figure 4.8   Interactions of cAMP and calcium in the control of steroidogenesis in the adrenal cortex. ACTH causes an increase in cAMP and thus activates protein kinase which phosphorylates a ribosomal component to stimulate the synthesis of a protein which promotes cholesterol sidechain cleavage; the protein kinase also activates cholesterol esterase, thus mobilizing steroid hormone precursor. There may also be an increase in the intracellular level of calcium which could stimulate steroidogenesis at several points. After Berridge, M. J. (1975) *Advances in Cyclic Nucleotide Research*, **6**, 1–98.

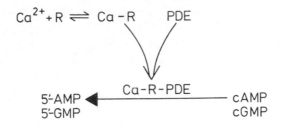

Figure 4.9   A tentative scheme for the activation of phosphodiesterase activity by intracellular calcium. R represents a calcium-dependent phosphoprotein regulator of phosphodiesterase (PDE).

problematical. For example, in the adrenal cortex, Ca^{++} seems to be involved at more than one step in ACTH action (figure 4.8). An optimum concentration of extracellular Ca^{++} is required for ACTH stimulation of adenylate cyclase. Additionally, while exogenous cAMP will activate steroidogenesis in the adrenal in the absence of extracellular Ca^{++}, the presence of Ca^{++} enhances the action of the nucleotide. Although there is evidence that Ca^{++} may also be involved in polypeptide chain elongation at the ribosomes, in general the role of Ca^{++} in the adrenal cortex remains unclear. In some other tissues, where Ca^{++} has been shown to be the primary second messenger, cAMP modulates the Ca^{++} signal. When cAMP is the primary second messenger, Ca^{++} could operate in a similar manner with regard to cAMP—perhaps by controlling the degradation of cAMP (or stimulating guanylate cyclase?). There is some evidence that Ca^{++}-binding proteins could act as activators of phosphodiesterase (figure 4.9) by analogy with the cAMP activation of cAMP-PrK. Such research is in its infancy and the scheme presented in figure 4.9 is largely speculative. The role of cGMP in cellular processes is also still not understood, but it has been proposed that cGMP could be an antagonist of the action of cAMP; in many tissues high levels of cAMP are associated with low levels of cGMP and vice versa. Clearly, a full understanding of second messenger actions must await the outcome of further research.

4.1.10   *Do peptide hormones enter their target cells?*
We have said that peptide or protein hormones do not need to enter their target cells to activate adenylate cyclase. Indeed, there is much evidence to support this view. The discovery of protein hormone receptors on the surfaces of target cells added weight to the "conventional wisdom" that proteins (hormones) could not easily pass through plasma membranes.

The short-term effects of peptide hormones (cAMP mediated responses) can be elicited even when the hormone is prevented from entering the cell. For example, the addition of ACTH to a suspension of adrenocortical cells will produce an increase in corticosteroid synthesis within about 3 min. This effect can be provoked when the ACTH is in a form covalently attached to very large molecules (e.g. dextrans) or even synthetic resin beads—which obviously could not pass through plasma membranes.

Such studies gave rise to the belief that because peptide hormones do not need to enter cells for some of their actions—they never do! Despite considerable inertia and disbelief on the part of many endocrinologists it is now clear that many protein and peptide hormones *do* enter their target cells. That this can occur is really not so surprising (perhaps with the benefit of hindsight). Phagocytosis is a primitive property retained by many cells. Several recent studies have shown that protein hormones gain access to the interiors of their target cells ("*internalization*") by a similar mechanism—receptor-mediated endocytosis (figure 4.10).

There is good evidence that parathyroid hormone, growth hormone, insulin, prolactin and gonadotropins enter cells. Parathyroid hormone, for example, in one of its actions binds to receptors on renal cells, and activates adenylate cyclase; the hormone also enters the cells and becomes associated with the mitochondria, modifying ion transport functions in these organelles. Extraction of the intracellular hormone complex shows that it retains both its biological and immunochemical reactivity. Similar evidence has been obtained for other polypeptide hormones but their eventual location within the target cells varies from hormone to hormone.

These observations are important, and should lead us to ask what the hormones are doing in cells. Do the hormones enter cells to bring about their more long-term effects? Is further processing of the hormone involved—for example, by lysosomes? Do hormones take their receptors into cells? If so, is this for degradation of the receptors, the hormone, or both? The answers to these questions may hold the key to a full understanding of how polypeptide hormones work.

4.2 Steroid hormones

Most steroid hormones exert their primary influence by initiating *de novo* synthesis of specific proteins, presumably by acting at the level of genetic transcription. Quantitative and qualitative changes in RNA synthesis usually precede the steroid hormone stimulation of inducible protein synthesis. Indeed it has been shown that a number of steroids (sex steroids

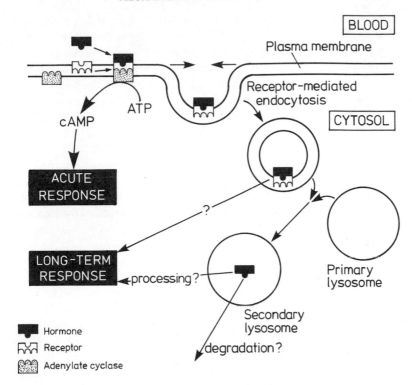

Figure 4.10 A scheme showing internalization of protein and peptide hormones by receptor-mediated endocytosis in target cells. Binding of hormone to the plasma membrane receptor provokes (i) cAMP formation, and acute intracellular responses, and (ii) endocytotic uptake of hormone (perhaps still attached to receptor), and longer-term responses.

in chicks and ecdysone in insects) induce a net increase in the specific mRNA molecules (coded for specific proteins) in their target cells. This brief description of their mechanism of action is too simple; steroid hormones which initiate growth and differentiation in their target tissues obviously act in a more complicated way, but the biochemical analysis of the complex processes involved in development is very difficult. Nevertheless, the production of specific proteins serves as a useful starting point for the analysis of steroid hormone action.

What is the evidence that steroids act on the nucleus at the level of genetic transcription? Ecdysone is a steroid hormone which initiates moulting in arthropods (§6.1.1). In the salivary glands of larval insects remarkable visible changes take place in the appearance of the "giant" or polytene chromosomes in response to ecdysone. These polytene chromosomes consist of numerous threads of chromatin lying side by side. Along their length a pattern of bands can be observed which represent sites of condensed DNA. At sites where the chromosomal material has unfolded or "puffed out", RNA synthesis is thought to be proceeding rapidly. Such sites, or chromosome puffs, would represent sites of transcription of genetic material (derepressed genes)—non-puffing segments of the chromosomes representing suppressed genes. Small doses of ecdysone (2×10^{-6} µg per animal) will induce a characteristic puff in salivary gland chromosomes of *Chironomus tentans* within 15–30 min of injection. This initial puff is followed by a second, 15–30 min later, and then by several more after a number of hours. The antibiotic, actinomycin D, which blocks DNA-dependant RNA synthesis, prevents the puff formation by ecdysone. Puromycin, which blocks protein synthesis in the cytoplasm at the translational level, does not prevent the two initial ecdysone-induced puffs, but does prevent the development of subsequent puffs. The later puffs thus depend on interactions of the earlier puffs with the cytoplasm, but the two early puffs must occur as a direct response to ecdysone and are central to the mechanism by which the steroid activates the cell.

Supportive evidence that steroids act at the nuclear level to control differential gene expression was indicated from observations that radioactively labelled steroids become localized in target cell nuclei; this is so for α-ecdysone in insect epidermal cells and aldosterone in rat kidney. Thus, steroid hormones enter their target cells. Indeed, experiments with ³H-oestradiol show that large amounts of hormone enter non-target tissues too. How, then, can steroid hormones be specific in their actions? A critical difference is that although non-target tissues take up steroids, they lose them more quickly than do target cells, suggesting that target tissues bind the hormone in some way and retard its exit.

4.2.1 *Steroid receptors*

There appears to be little if any regulation of steroid entry into cells. Steroids, because of their lipid nature, readily diffuse across the plasma membrane from the blood and enter most cells. Only in target cells, however, are there specific receptors which reversibly bind the steroids and, in so doing, lead to the eventual expression of the hormone's biological activity. Receptors for ecdysone have not been studied and most of the detailed information of steroid hormone action comes from studies of their cytoplasmic receptors in the female reproductive tracts of chickens and rats. In particular, it is known that the vagina, uterus and oviduct contain oestrogen receptors. These have a high affinity for the hormone and the binding characteristics correlate well with the physiological concentrations found in the blood. Antagonists of binding to these cytoplasmic receptors are also antagonistic to steroid hormone action and, in general, specificity of binding matches specificity of action; cytoplasmic receptors for steroid hormones are thus an integral part of their action. Considerable research has been centred on finding and characterizing such receptors. In particular, the localization of cytosolic fractions (containing bound radioactively labelled steroid hormone) has been studied extensively using sucrose gradient centrifugation. Although estimates of the size of cytoplasmic receptors from such studies vary, a theory of steroid hormone action has evolved which suggests that binding to the cytoplasmic receptor is followed by a configurational change during translocation into the nucleus. Here, binding to a further receptor occurs to initiate genetic transcription. The change in configuration of the hormone-receptor complex in the cytosol was inferred from changes in sedimentation coefficient (with sucrose density gradient) but it is possible that such changes are artefacts of the extraction procedures. Indeed, it has been shown that the sedimentation coefficient of the oestrogen receptors from rat uterus is variable and can be influenced considerably by the ionic strength of the sucrose gradient, the concentration of receptor protein, the presence of other proteins from the tissue or tissue components, and the presence of polyanions. It is possible therefore that there may be no real difference between the oestrogen receptors in the cytoplasm and in the nucleus (figure 4.11).

What evidence is there that the cytoplasmic receptors move into the nuclear compartment? First, oestrogen receptors are always present in the cytoplasm, but in the nucleus they are found only after oestrogen treatment. Second, the concentration of oestrogen receptors in the cytoplasm decreases after hormone application. For example, although the concentration of receptors varies during the reproductive cycle, a large dose of oestrogen causes a rapid depletion of cytoplasmic receptors (to 10% of initial value) which correlates with the appearance of receptors in the nucleus (and, of course, the rapid appearance of injected radiolabelled hormone in the nucleus). Thus, although the evidence is indirect, the translocation of the hormone receptor complex from the cytoplasm into the nucleus is generally accepted.

The chick oviduct responds to oestrogen treatment by growth, differentiation, and secretion of ovalbumin. If oestrogen treatment is discontinued, the rate of ovalbumin synthesis drops and after 12 days is only

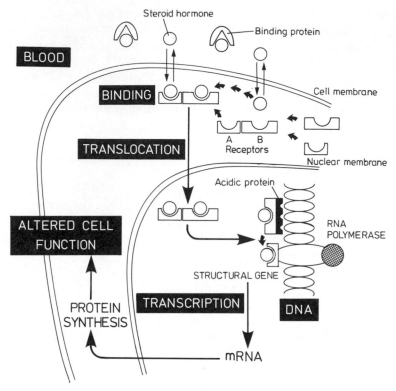

Figure 4.11 A tentative model for steroid hormone action based on a study of the progesterone receptors in chick oviduct. After Schrader, W. T. and O'Malley, B. W., in *Hormone Receptors* (D. M. Klachko, L. R. Forte and J. M. Franz, eds.) 109–130, Plenum Press, N.Y., 1978.

1 % of the hormonally-stimulated rate. If either oestrogen or progesterone are now given, there is a rapid increase in ovalbumin synthesis. Thus, although prior to oestrogen treatment progesterone cannot induce ovalbumin synthesis, in oviducts which have been "primed" by oestrogens, progesterone mimics this oestrogenic action. In fact, oestrogens cause the appearance of progesterone receptors in the oviductal cytoplasm. When oestrogen and progesterone are administered together, to chicks which had earlier received oestrogen treatment (now withdrawn for several days), their effects on RNA synthesis are not additive; this suggests that these two steroids act at identical nuclear sites to initiate transcription. The progesterone stimulation of genetic transcription has been used successfully as a model for studies on steroid hormone action by Professor

B. W. O'Malley and his colleagues in Houston, Texas. They have purified the progesterone receptor in chick oviduct and studied its role in the initiation of transcription. A scheme for this is presented in figure 4.11.

4.2.2   Nuclear acceptors

It is thought that the hormone-receptor complex enters the nucleus and binds to some component(s) of the chromatin. O'Malley and colleagues believe that the specificity of binding of the progesterone-receptor complex to chromatin lies in the non-histone, acidic proteins. They concluded this from an elegant series of experiments involving hybridization of chromatin proteins:

(i)   Binding of a radioactively labelled progesterone-receptor complex to intact erythrocyte (i.e. non-target) chromatin was negligible compared with that to chromatin from the oviduct.
(ii)   Hybrid chromatins made of DNA from erythrocytes and a histone-acidic protein fraction from oviduct showed binding comparable to that of intact (or reconstituted) oviduct chromatin.
(iii)   Hybrids of DNA from oviducts with a histone-acidic protein fraction from erythrocytes showed poor binding comparable to that with intact erythrocyte chromatin (figure 4.12).

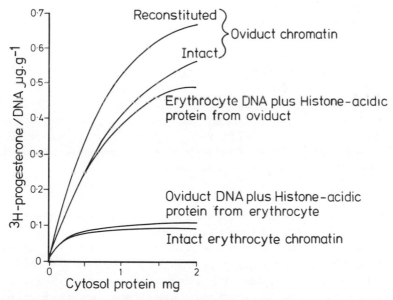

Figure 4.12   Binding of labelled oviduct progesterone-receptor complex to intact and reconstituted chick chromatin. After Spelsberg, T. C., *et al.*, (1971) *J. Biol. Chem.*, **246**, 4188–4197.

These workers have purified the progesterone-receptor complex to homogeneity and shown that it consists of A (110 000 molecular weight) and B (117 000 molecular weight) subunits. Subunit A binds to pure DNA but poorly to chromatin, whereas B binds to non-histone protein DNA complexes of oviduct chromatin but not to pure DNA. These observations have led to the suggestion that the A subunit could be the actual gene regulatory protein, and the B subunit could specify where the A subunit is to localize. In fact, in the absence of the B subunit, A can stimulate transcription in a cell-free *in vitro* system, but only at concentrations 10–50 fold higher than that required for the intact progesterone-receptor complex. Subunit B is without activity in this situation. It is thought that the A subunit is capable of destabilizing a portion of the chromatin-DNA identified by the B subunit so that new sites are available for RNA polymerase, allowing mRNA synthesis. These observations are consistent with the model presented in figure 4.11 but other models are currently under consideration. It is possible for example, that oestrogens (and other steroids?) act at more than one intracellular site. In particular, there is evidence that the half-life of mRNA coded for ovalbumin is only 3 h following oestrogen withdrawal, compared with about 30 h in the continued presence of the hormone. Clearly, much remains to be understood concerning the mechanism of action of the steroid-receptor complex in the nucleus.

The juvenile hormone of insects, although not a steroid (§ 2.2.3), deserves some mention here. It appears to act by influencing gene expression both in larvae (in regulating development) and in adult insects (inducing vitellogenesis). Specific cytoplasmic receptors have not been described for juvenile hormones but high affinity binding sites are found in epidermal nuclei at certain stages. More research into receptors for juvenile hormones (and for ecdysone) is required, but we can speculate that the general mode of action of these hormones in insects is similar to that outlined for vertebrate steroid hormones.

4.2.3   *Extra-nuclear actions*

Several effects of steroid hormones occur within seconds of their interaction with target cells and are insensitive to actinomycin D. It would seem, therefore, that transcription is not involved and the scheme presented in figure 4.11 is not applicable to these rapidly elicited effects. In particular, oestrogens appear to affect membrane permeability, and aldosterone stimulates potassium excretion by processes which cannot immediately involve a stimulation of *de novo* protein synthesis, but the exact mechanisms are uncertain.

Steroid hormones are also known to be concerned with differentiation of the brain (see §7.1), and oestrogen receptors in the hypothalamic neurones appear also to be involved in controlling sexual behaviour and aggression. Circulating androgens may be metabolized in these neurones to form oestrogens (figure 7.6), and thus become capable of binding to such oestrogen receptors to modulate behaviour. Interestingly, some antiandrogens, such as cyproterone acetate, inhibit the enzymes involved in this conversion. Drugs like this are used to ameliorate some forms of pathological hypersexuality in human males.

Some of the metabolic effects of testosterone can be mimicked by exogenous cAMP but this nucleotide cannot induce specific protein synthesis nor the morphogenetic effects of the steroid. Cyclic AMP will stimulate tyrosine transaminase in the liver of rats, thus mimicking glucocorticoid action, but when the nucleotide is added together with cortisol their effects are additive. It would seem, therefore, that they act by separate mechanisms.

On the other hand, oestrogens appear to cause a rapid increase in intracellular concentration of cAMP in rat uterus but the effect is probably caused by the oestrogen-induced release of catecholamines. More long-term effects of steroids on cyclic nucleotides are known. For example, corticosteroids are thought to increase the responsiveness of adipose tissue to catecholamines and growth hormone by a mechanism which involves protein synthesis (it is sensitive to actinomycin D)—perhaps by stimulating the synthesis of adenylate cyclase.

4.3 Thyroid hormones

Thyroid hormones affect growth, development and metabolic activity in most cells. They stimulate oxygen consumption, affect Na^+/K^+ ATP-ase activity, increase RNA synthesis, and have morphogenetic effects which are especially prominent in some lower vertebrates (§ 7.7.1). A further, more specific, action is the maintenance of normal growth hormone content in the pituitary: in the absence of thyroid hormone, the pituitary content of growth hormone declines rapidly. Despite considerable interest and research, the details of thyroid hormone action are still poorly understood.

Early hypotheses advanced concerning the site of thyroid hormone action favoured two possibilities; a direct effect on the nucleus or a direct interaction of the hormones with extranuclear organelles, particularly the mitochondria. A third possibility is, of course, a combination of these (figure 4.13).

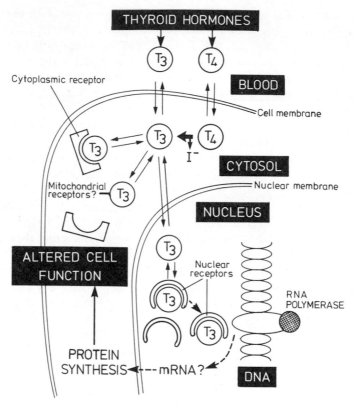

Figure 4.13   A tentative scheme for the action of thyroid hormones.

T_3 may be the active thyroid hormone, and T_4 could represent a prohormone. T_3 is more potent and binds more avidly to nuclear and mitochondrial receptors than T_4. Binding sites for thyroxine have been demonstrated in the nucleus (possibly located in the chromatin), on cytoplasmic proteins, and in mitochondria. The nuclear binding sites are high affinity, low capacity receptors whilst the cytoplasmic sites appear to be non-specific and have low affinity and high capacity. Interestingly, mitochondria appear to contain a large number of non-specific hormone-binding sites but a smaller number of high affinity, limited capacity sites. These latter sites can be demonstrated only after partial purification of the mitochondrial membrane protein and are thought to be specific receptors (figure 4.13).

CHAPTER FIVE

METABOLISM

5.1 Hormones and the gut

The digestive tract of most animals is, in effect, a tube running from mouth to anus; it is lined with an epithelium which secretes digestive enzymes and absorbs the products of digestion. As food material enters the gut and traverses its length, a large number of physiological events involving muscular activity and glandular secretion must be coordinated to ensure the efficient digestion, absorption and assimilation of the various chemical components of the diet. Clearly, the speed of transport through the tract, the nature and timing of the appropriate enzyme release, and the physico-chemical environment created within the intestinal lumen are all import-ant in determining this end. In invertebrates, the role of the endocrine system in regulating these events has not been explored fully and may be very limited or, in some groups, absent; but the presence of chemicals in the food, or in the products of digestion, initiates or modulates feeding behaviour and influences digestive activity. These chemicals act rather as secretagogues in that they exert a local action as messengers by stimu-lating receptors associated with the feeding apparatus or the intestinal epithelium to initiate a direct and appropriate response to their presence. In *Hydra*, for example, glutathione, released from injured prey, induces an elaborate series of feeding movements. In higher invertebrates, the presence of sugars in the environment may exert similar effects, e.g. in the freshwater snail, *Lymnaea*, glucose solutions will increase the rate of radula movement; in blowflies and butterflies, a reflex extension of the proboscis is elicited by tarsal (the penultimate part of each leg) contact with sugar solutions. Additionally, it is known that in those invertebrates where

79

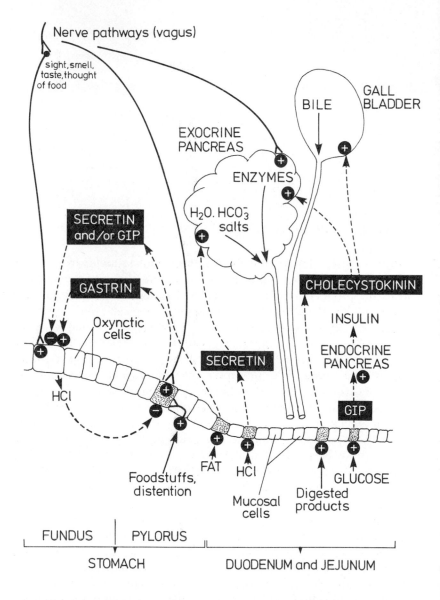

Figure 5.1 The role of hormones in controlling gastric acid secretion, pancreatic secretion of salts and enzymes, and the contraction of the gall bladder. After Bentley, P. J., in *Comparative Vertebrate Endocrinology*, Cambridge University Press, 175, 1976.

extracellular digestion occurs (many invertebrates rely largely on intra-cellular digestion) the qualitative and quantitative control of digestive enzyme secretion may be via the secretagogues in the diet.

In vertebrates a complex system of endocrine control has evolved whereby the gastrointestinal tract releases hormones into the blood in response to secretagogues present in the lumen. These hormones released from one part of the tract elicit muscular or secretory responses in another part (figure 5.1). The combined action of the autonomic nervous system and humoral reflex arcs in controlling the digestive system is best understood in mammals; we shall concern ourselves with this group only, but although direct evidence is often lacking, it is assumed that the situation is similar in lower vertebrates.

5.1.1 *Gastrin*

The process of eating (or its anticipation) leads to a rapid secretion of saliva via a reflex pathway of the autonomic nervous system. The endocrine system is not involved. In chapter 1 we discussed the relative virtues of nervous and endocrine control, and here, in the control of salivary gland function, we see again that the nervous system controls transient processes which must occur rapidly when they are needed. However, the stimulation of the taste buds (or visual or olfactory stimuli) also initiates via the vagus nerve the release of a hormone, gastrin, from the pyloric region of the stomach. The vagal innervation of the stomach also stimulates the cells of gastric mucosa to produce a gastric juice rich in the enzyme pepsin, and additionally it sensitizes these cells to gastrin; they thus release hydrochloric acid in response to the hormone, creating a low pH within the stomach suitable for peptic digestion. Partially digested protein in the stomach may be a strong stimulus for further gastrin release via a local nervous mechanism (figure 5.1). The overall control of gastrin release is exerted by a closed loop mechanism whereby excess acid in the stomach inhibits further release of hormone. Other hormones, such as secretin and GIP (glucose-dependent insulin-releasing peptide) from the duodenum, may also play a role in inhibiting gastrin release.

Three molecular forms of the gastrin peptide have been isolated which are all identical in their C-terminal portions (figure 2.7) but differ in chain length; it is perhaps not surprising therefore that C-terminal integrity is essential for activity. Additional larger forms of gastrin ("big" and "big-big" gastrin) are also found in tissue and blood but their physiological significance is uncertain. The distribution of gastrin in non-mammalian vertebrates has not been explored systematically and, despite its existence in birds and teleosts, only in these higher tetrapods has its characteristic physiological action been shown.

The availability of synthetic gastrin has allowed the source of the hormone to be demonstrated. Antibodies raised against a synthetic human gastrin can be labelled with fluorescein and used to locate cells in the pyloric region of the stomach; these cells react with the fluorescein-labelled antibody in histological sections of the stomach and can be identified by the fluorescent precipitate within their cytoplasm. Interestingly, the same cells show formalin-induced fluorescence—a characteristic of APUD cells (§ 1.6).

5.1.2   Secretin

The presence of hydrochloric acid in the intestinal lumen initiates the release of another peptide hormone, secretin. This hormone belongs to a family of peptides as we have mentioned briefly in a previous discussion (see § 2.2.2). Included in this family are two peptides, GIP (glucose-dependent insulin-releasing peptide) and VIP (vasoactive intestinal peptide), whose physiological functions are not well understood (see below). The close similarities in the structures of these peptides are shown in figure 5.2. Secretin stimulates the secretion of bicarbonate by the exocrine pancreas and the biliary tract, and its major effect is therefore to neutralize the acid chyme (another closed loop feedback system). Similar mechanisms probably operate in lower vertebrates because secretin-like peptides have been found in most groups.

5.1.3   Cholecystokinin

The mucosal cells in the upper regions of the intestine release another peptide hormone, cholecystokinin (figure 2.7), in response to the presence of digested fat or protein in the intestinal lumen (fatty acids of 10 or more carbon atoms and the amino acids tryptophan and phenylalanine are most effective). This hormone stimulates pancreatic secretion (the zymogens of the powerful proteases—trypsins and chymotrypsins—and amylases and lipases) and contraction of the gall bladder, and it also inhibits gastric emptying. These actions can be considered part of short feedback loops because they facilitate digestion (neutralizing acid and emulsifying fats) and absorption of the foods that cause the hormone's release.

Cholecystokinin and secretin are potentiative synergists; each augments the primary actions of the other. It may be that the small amounts of secretin released under natural feeding conditions would have little effect if

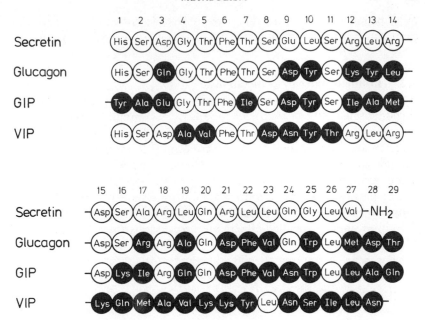

Figure 5.2 Amino acid sequences of secretin and the homologous peptides glucagon, GIP and VIP. Identities different from those of secretin are shown by the dark circles. GIP has 43 residues but only the amino terminal 29 are shown. From Grossman, M. I., in *Peptide Hormones* (J. A. Parsons, ed.) Macmillan Press, 108, 1976.

it were not for the potentiative effect of cholecystokinin (which is released in larger amounts).

5.1.4 Other intestinal hormones and candidate hormones

Although a large number of peptides have been identified in the intestinal mucosa and can be shown to have various effects on digestive processes, their physiological significance is not always clear. We shall mention only two such peptides, GIP and VIP (figure 5.2).

GIP is released after a carbohydrate-rich meal, and its primary action may be to elicit insulin release from the endocrine pancreas. It may also inhibit gastric motility and gastric secretion. VIP has a relaxing effect on smooth muscle and has some secretin-like properties, but its physiological function is unclear. We mention VIP here because of its chemical structure (figure 5.2) and its apparently wide distribution in the body; it is present in the intestinal mucosa, the endocrine pancreas, and the brain. VIP and the other peptides found in the intestine are best described for the present as candidate hormones which may, after further study, qualify as hormones.

5.2 Hormones and energy metabolism

Animals may oxidize a variety of substances for energy, but in general, carbohydrates and fats are the major and most commonly used fuels. With only minor exceptions, similar biochemical pathways are employed by invertebrates and vertebrates to generate ATP from carbohydrate or fat catabolism. We will examine the mechanisms by which these fuels are made available in sufficient quantity to support energy metabolism, paying particular attention to the endocrine mechanisms controlling their supply during exercise or starvation.

In invertebrates, detailed information concerning the endocrine control of carbohydrate and fat metabolism is available only for insects. The development of immunochemical methods for detecting and assaying vertebrate hormones such as insulin, glucagon and gastrin has prompted an upsurge of publications which suggest that invertebrates possess (and use) such hormones. In fact these observations show only that some invertebrates possess peptides or (bits of?) proteins which have perhaps limited structural affinities with vertebrate peptides. Some invertebrates respond pharmacologically to vertebrate peptides (and vice versa), but in few studies is there any clear indication that these immuno-reactive invertebrate proteins are released into the blood to act as hormones. However, more established and thorough endocrinological approaches have shown that insects possess hormones with hyperglycaemic, hypo-glycaemic, hyperlipaemic and hypolipaemic activities. For these reasons we will restrict our discussion of invertebrate hormones to those of insects, in particular the locust, and draw comparisons with what is known of the actions of vertebrate (and particularly mammalian) hormones with similar properties.

5.2.1 *Physiological responses to exercise and starvation*

At first sight, it may appear surprising that the general metabolic responses to exercise and starvation (figure 5.3) are similar, but the requirements of animals in both situations are essentially the same.

Whereas most tissues can obtain their energy requirement by the oxidation of a variety of fuels, this is not so in the nervous system, red blood cells, kidney medulla or testis; these tissues have an obligatory and continuing requirement for glucose and therefore the body's carbohydrate

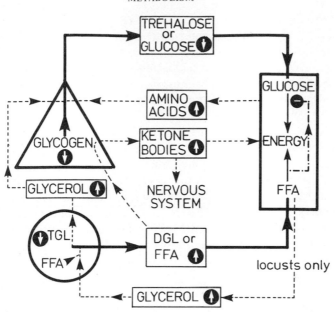

Figure 5.3 Schematic summary of the metabolic events during starvation and exercise. Metabolic pathways are shown ——▶, primary; – – –▶, secondary. Feedback is shown —·—·—▶. ⬆ = increase, ⬇ = decrease. TGL = triacylglycerol; DGL = diacylglycerol; FFA = free fatty acid. ⊖ = inhibition. △ = liver; ◯ – adipose tissue; ☐ = muscle.

stores must be conserved particularly for their use, especially during times of relative lack—during exercise and starvation. This is made possible by a change in the type of fuel used, which is undergone by most tissues under these conditions. In general, those tissues which can oxidize fat do so, thus sparing glucose.

It should be clear from figure 5.3 that the responses of vertebrates and insects to starvation and exercise are remarkably similar, although some differences exist. First, although insects store fats as triacylglycerol (TGL) as in vertebrates, they mobilize them in the form of diacylglycerol (DGL) rather than FFA (free or non-esterified fatty acids) as in vertebrates. The fate of the glycerol released when TGL is hydrolyzed (lipolysis) therefore differs in the two groups: in insects it can be used for re-esterification of FFA rather than for gluconeogenesis as in vertebrates. Second, the major blood carbohydrate in insects is usually trehalose (a disaccharide of glucose) which is often present in high concentration (up to 4 g %), whereas free glucose concentrations are comparable with those in vertebrates (around 50–150 mg %). Third, insects have no recognizable separate liver or adipose tissue, and the fat body appears to fulfil many of the functions of both of these vertebrate tissues. Consequently, in figure 5.8 the fat body is represented as a combination of liver and adipose tissue but it should not be assumed that its various functions are all undertaken by any single cell type.

A fundamental aspect of the scheme presented in figure 5.3 is the inhibition of glucose utilization during periods of increased fatty acid or ketone body oxidation. The glucose-fatty acid cycle theory, proposed by Professor P. J. Randle and his colleagues, attempts to explain the decreased rate of glucose utilization in muscles and nervous tissue (during starvation or prolonged exercise) by an inhibition of phosphofructokinase by citrate (see figure 5.4). The citrate concentration in the cytosol of muscle (and liver) is known to be much more variable than in the mitochondria, and can change more than 60-fold (between $30 \mu M$ and $2 mM$) under different metabolic conditions. Thus citrate could contribute to the regulation of phosphofructokinase (and hence glycolysis). This theory may be applicable to vertebrates and perhaps some invertebrates, but phosphofructokinase from a variety of insect tissues is insensitive to citrate, and the inhibition of glycolysis may operate instead through aldolase (which is sensitive to citrate, at least in locusts).

One further aspect of the scheme presented in figure 5.3 is the utilization of glycerol and amino acids such as alanine (derived from proteolysis of skeletal muscle) for gluconeogenesis. During starvation, the carbohydrate reserves of the body in man, for example, would satisfy the demand for glucose for only about 12 h. Man can survive starvation for several months; during this period, therefore, glucose must be synthesized from non-carbohydrate precursors. This gluconeogenesis occurs principally in the liver and kidney medulla, but at a rate which is sufficient to supply the brain, for example, with only a fraction of its normal requirement of glucose. However, many of the molecules of acetyl CoA formed in the liver by the partial oxidation of long-chain fatty acids are condensed and transported from the liver, two at a time, as ketone bodies—acetoacetate and β-hydroxybutyrate. These are readily oxidized by muscle during the early stages of starvation and eventually, as starvation persists, by the brain, where they provide the major proportion of the energy supply and accordingly displace glucose utilization. The decreased demand for glucose and increased oxidation of fatty acids in the muscles, together with the ability of ketone bodies to supplement the fuel supply of the nervous

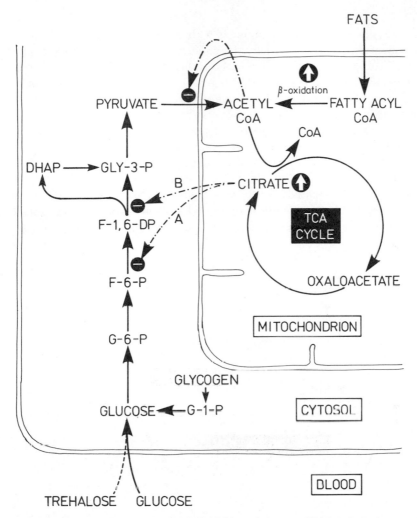

Figure 5.4 A proposed mechanism for the inhibition of glucose utilization during increased fatty acid oxidation. In vertebrates, inhibition of glycolysis would occur at phosphofructo-kinase, A, but in insects it could be at aldolase, B. G-1-P, glucose-1-phosphate; G-6-P, glucose-6-phosphate; F-6-P, fructose-6-phosphate; F-1,6-DP, fructose-1,6-diphosphate; GLY-3-P, glycerol-3-phosphate; DHAP, dihydroxyacetone phosphate.

system, therefore represent important physiological mechanisms whereby excessive proteolysis of the skeletal muscles is delayed so that the animal can remain active and able to capture or forage for food.

5.2.2   *The fed state*

Our main concern in this chapter is with starvation and exercise but it is pertinent first to discuss briefly the endocrinological processes associated with feeding. Very little is known about this in locusts. Feeding is a strong stimulus for the release of cerebral neurosecretion in insects, and blood diglyceride in starved locusts falls rapidly to normal fed values within 6 h of being given grass; there is, however, no clear evidence of any hormonal involvement in this response and it may be a direct effect of increased glucose availability allowing triglyceride synthesis (see figure 5.5).

In mammals, the ingestion of a mixed meal is followed by the rapid release of insulin. Contrary to earlier concepts, this is probably not due directly to an increased level of blood glucose after absorption from the intestine, but (in anticipation of such an event) is most likely due to stimulation of insulin release by GIP from the upper small intestine (see

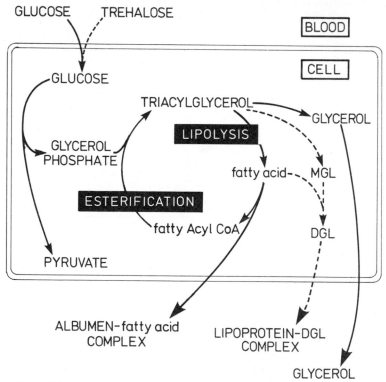

Figure 5.5   The triacylglycerol-fatty acid cycle. The broken lines represent the situation in insects.

figure 5.1). Thus, the immediate post-prandial period is characterized by high titres of insulin which trigger increased protein uptake and storage of carbohydrate and fat. This is followed by a period characterized by the appearance of growth hormone in the plasma which, at modest insulin titres, stimulates biosynthetic and growth processes which utilize carbohydrate and amino acids. Thus increased fatty acid oxidation in peripheral tissues spares carbohydrate to some extent during this period. Finally, as the time after the meal becomes greater, insulin titres fall, and in the presence of growth hormone (and other lipolytic hormones), fatty acid oxidation predominates over that of glucose until the next meal. If the next meal is not readily forthcoming, then starvation conditions ensue.

5.2.3 *Hormonal mechanisms during starvation*
Starvation in insects During fasting, insects consume first the small reserves of glycogen, but fat is always the major reserve substance that is drawn upon during long term starvation. Thus blood and tissue carbohydrates decrease and the concentration of blood lipid is maintained or increases at the expense of stored TGL. In many insects, proteolysis may support gluconeogenesis but this has received little detailed study. There is no convincing evidence that insects (or indeed any animals) can synthesize carbohydrate from fat, but glycerol, released during fat degradation, can be converted to trehalose or glycogen. Formation of ketone bodies by the fat body is known to increase in starved locusts but this appears not to have been studied in other insects.

Although trehalose is the major blood sugar in most insects, free glucose is present in the blood, in variable but comparable concentrations to those found in mammals (but relatively low compared with those of trehalose), and appears to be maintained during starvation at a basal level. In the locust, blood trehalose concentrations are maintained only for the first few hours of starvation (at the expense of glycogen in the fat body and gut but not that in the flight muscles) and fall steadily during 5 days of starvation. The concentration of DGL in the blood is maintained for the first two days of starvation but then increases steadily so that after 5 days it may have increased by 300%. The mechanism by which hyperlipaemia occurs during starvation in locusts is uncertain but appears not to be hormonal. If a triacylglycerol/fatty acid cycle similar to that in vertebrate adipose tissue (figure 5.5) operates in locusts, then it is possible to explain how these changes during starvation could occur independently of hormones; as the level of blood glucose decreases, the rate of entry of glucose into the fat body would drop, the rate of glycolysis would decrease and lower the glycerol phosphate content. Consequently, the rate of esterification would decrease (see figure 5.5), thus increasing the mobilization of DGL since lipolysis would be unaffected. Conversely, a rise in blood carbohydrate would cause a decrease in lipid mobilization—an effect which can be demonstrated when trehalose is injected into starved locusts. Such a mechanism as is depicted in figure 5.5 could therefore explain some of the observed metabolic changes in locusts during starvation, but it may eventually be shown that hormones are involved.

Gluconeogenesis in locusts has not been studied but the amino acid content of the blood increases during starvation, and, if amino acids are used for gluconeogenesis in the fat body, this may partly account for the maintenance of blood glucose. Ketone body formation also increases during starvation, but utilization by the fat body and flight muscles decreases, while that by the testes remains unchanged. Unfortunately,

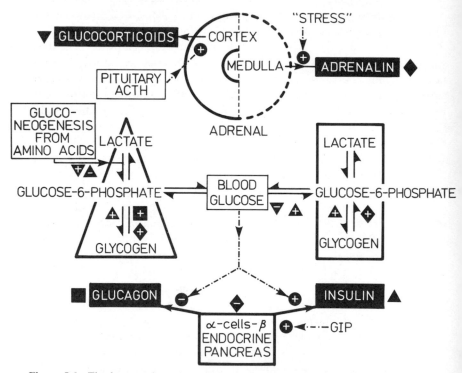

Figure 5.6 The hormonal regulation of blood glucose concentration in mammals. The influence of hormones is shown by the signs (positive for stimulation, negative for inhibition) in the appropriate symbol for each hormone. For other symbols see figure 5.3.

ketone body utilization by insect nervous tissue has not been investigated, so we can only guess at the significance of these metabolic changes during starvation, and imagine that their close parallels with those in vertebrates represent common functions.

Starvation in vertebrates In higher animals, blood glucose concentrations are regulated by a sophisticated array of hormones (figure 5.6). These normally do not allow the blood glucose concentrations to fall by more than about 30% and so lipid mobilization is necessarily regulated by hormones. Thus mobilization of fatty acids can be brought about in response to conditions which are unrelated to large fluctuations in blood glucose.

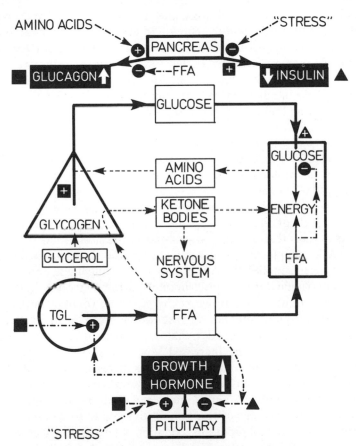

Figure 5.7 The endocrine control of metabolism during starvation or exercise in vertebrates. For explanation of symbols see figures 5.3 and 5.6.

Figure 5.7 summarises in a simple manner the metabolic and hormonal events occurring during starvation in higher vertebrates. As the levels of circulating insulin fall, muscle proteolysis outweighs synthesis, certain amino acids are metabolized in the muscle and those which are glucogenic (such as alanine) are released. The low levels of insulin, and normal or high glucagon titres, direct the liver towards glucose synthesis, the energy for which is met by hepatic oxidation of fat. A decrease in insulin titre reduces lipogenesis (see figure 5.5) and causes increased release of fatty acid from adipose tissue; other hormones are also involved in promoting lipolysis, including glucocorticoids, growth hormone and glucagon. The hyper-lipaemic properties of glucagon are very variable between vertebrate species but in man, birds and dogs, glucagon is markedly hyperlipaemic and glucagon titre is known to increase in fasting humans. On the other hand, an increase in growth hormone titre could also be important during starvation in mammals (except perhaps the rat) since, in the presence of glucocorticoids, the hormone stimulates lipolysis, and potentiates the cAMP-response of adipose tissue to catecholamines—which may also be important during the early stages of starvation.

5.2.4   *Hormonal mechanisms during exercise*
Flight in insects   For some exercise, muscle glycogen provides sufficient energy. But for prolonged activities, animals must make available in the blood supply to the muscles either an adequate supply of existing fuel or an alternative. For example, in blowflies, which rely entirely on carbo-hydrate as fuel for flight activity, the release of a hypertrehalosaemic hormone ensures that a steady state concentration of blood trehalose is maintained to supply energy to the flight muscles. In cockroaches, flight muscle glycogen supplies 85 % of the fuel used during flight, and release of hypertrehalosaemic hormone does not appear to be involved in the flight metabolism of these insects; however this hormone could be important in maintaining adequate supplies of fuel for enforced (walking) activity. During flight in locusts, blood trehalose is used initially by the flight muscles but eventually the increased amounts of DGL in the blood become the predominant source of fuel. This increase in concentration of DGL in the blood is caused by the release of adipokinetic hormone (AKH) from the corpora cardiaca. This stimulates a TGL lipase in the fat body (and a monoacylglycerol acyltransferase, figure 5.8) to cause release of DGL into the blood, and promotes oxidation of fatty acids (liberated from the DGL) in the flight muscles. The decrease in trehalose utilization by the flight muscles correlates with their increased oxidation of fatty acids (see

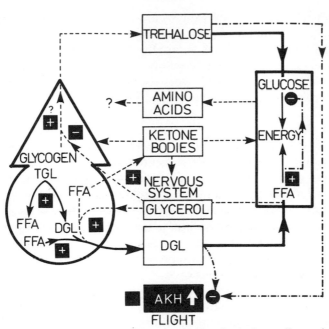

Figure 5.8 The endocrine control of flight metabolism in the locust. For explanation of symbols see figures 5.3 and 5.6.

figure 5.8). AKH also stimulates ketone body production in the fat body and favours incorporation of glycerol into blood DGL rather than into trehalose (figure 5.8). Thus, in the locust, the involvement of AKH in prolonged flight ensures that carbohydrate reserves are conserved for utilization by those tissues which require it continuously.

Exercise in vertebrates The hormonal changes which occur during exercise in vertebrates are essentially similar to those during starvation and are represented in figure 5.7. The plasma levels of insulin decrease, whereas those of adrenalin, growth hormone, glucocorticoids and glucagon increase. These hormonal changes result in increased rates of gluconeogenesis in the liver (see §4.1.7), lipolysis in the adipose tissue (which increases the plasma levels of FFA and glycerol), glycogenolysis in the liver, and decreased demand for glucose (and increased utilization of fatty acids) in the muscles. The changes are thus very similar to those in starvation, but occur more rapidly.

It has been suggested recently that, in man at least, the peripheral tissues (probably the vascular endothelium) are capable of binding insulin non-specifically in significant amounts which can be released rapidly during the initial stages of exercise. Such a rapid transient supply of insulin to the muscles at the start of exercise could be very important in the control of energy metabolism but more work is needed in this area before its significance can be assessed fully.

5.2.5 *Diabetes mellitus*

Finally, no discussion of the role of insulin and the control of metabolism would be complete without a brief mention of diabetes. About 2 % of the population of Western Europe and North America (perhaps 10 million people) suffer from this condition—a disease characterized by high blood glucose levels (hyperglycaemia). Often in diabetics there is an absence of circulating insulin, due to some fault in the pancreatic β-cells (or a reduced number of these cells), but in many cases insulin levels are normal or above average. These latter cases must represent a reduced ability of the tissues either to recognize the hormone (at the receptor level) or to respond at the intracellular level. Whichever is the cause of diabetes, the effects are clear; after a meal the rates of intestinal absorption and entry into the blood of carbohydrate, amino acids and fat (which are independent of insulin) will exceed those of the peripheral uptake of all fuels (which are insulin dependent). In a modest diabetic condition, insulin levels (or efficacy) may be sufficient to suppress ketogenesis and gluconeogenesis but insufficient to facilitate glucose entry into muscle and adipose tissue. Severe hyper-glycaemia may occur, glucose will be voided in the final urine (the maximum rate of renal reabsorption of glucose will be inadequate), dehydration will ensue and this may lead to hyperosmolar coma. If the diabetes is severe, then proteolysis of muscle will provide the liver with more and more glucogenic substrate, and gluconeogenesis will proceed rapidly. FFA levels in the blood will also be elevated, as lipolysis proceeds unrestrained. The influx of FFA into the liver will favour ketogenesis and eventually the concentration of ketone bodies in the blood will increase to dangerous levels; the pH buffering of the blood will be affected and ketoacidosis ensue. Diabetes is also associated with secondary changes in the secretion of cortisol, glucagon, growth hormone and catecholamines (all lipolytic in their effects) that aggravate the insulin deficiency. For many sufferers all the biochemical and hormonal changes can usually be restored to near normal with insulin treatment.

CHAPTER SIX

SKIN AND SKELETON

COLLECTIVELY, THE SKIN AND ASSOCIATED STRUCTURES COMPRISE THE integument, and form the major interface between the animal and its external environment. Not surprisingly, the integument shows great variety in anatomy and physiology according to habitat and lifestyle. It may be very thick and waterproof in some animals, yet very thin in others. Localized areas of the integument may have specialized functions. They may, for example, be transparent where they cover light sensitive areas, or they may form gills or cuticular flaps for gas exchange and ion transport. Animals which live a concealed existence in soil or as endoparasites are often colourless, or show colours determined either by the compounds used in the hardening of the skin or by the materials they eat (which can be seen through the skin). Most other animals are coloured either for camouflage or display and, with the exception of insects, commonly possess pigment-bearing ectodermal cells beneath the epidermis, called chromatophores. In all animals the integument has a skeletal function ranging from simple containment to the provision of a rigid exoskeleton in the arthropods. Many of these aspects of integument function are governed by hormones, and some of the more important ones will be discussed in this chapter.

6.1 Hormones and moulting
The integument is often subject to abrasion. It may be renewed more or less continuously, as is common in mammals, for example, or the whole skin may be shed and renewed at intervals varying from a few days in many amphibia and arthropods, to several months in reptiles. Many

95

mammals and birds show changes in the skin appendages (hairs and feathers) related to breeding or seasonal cycles. These processes, either the shedding of the entire skin or only of its appendages, are commonly referred to as moulting; the term clearly encompasses a wide and varied range of events in the integument.

6.1.1 *Arthropods*

Many invertebrates shed their skin but hormonal control has been investigated in detail only in arthropods where the rigid external skeleton limits the size of the animal; a dramatic increase in size and, therefore, the overt expression of growth during each intermoult stage (= instar), is possible only at ecdysis, when the cuticle is shed and the new cuticle is expanded. Ecdysis and the deposition of new cuticle are under hormonal control.

Insects The timing of the moult and the formation of new cuticle can be initiated by a variety of stimuli. In *Rhodnius*, for example, feeding is of prime importance; the bug takes one blood meal each instar and moults after a fixed period. The ingested blood may be 2–3 times the insect's own weight. Signals from stretch receptors in the distended abdomen travel via the ventral nerve cord to activate the cerebral neurosecretory cells. Brain hormone (ecdysiotropin) released from the corpus cardiacum acts on the prothoracic glands (figure 6.1) but release of brain hormone must continue for a number of days to fully activate the glands. This is called the critical period, and during this time removal of the cerebral neurosecretory cells prevents moulting. After the critical period, however, the prothoracic glands synthesize ecdysone independently of the brain's influence; removal of the neurosecretory cells is then without effect. A similar system operates in other insects but the cerebral neurosecretory cells are activated by a variety of stimuli in addition to feeding.

The action of ecdysteroids Prothoracic glands cultured *in vitro* release α-ecdysone, but in the intact insect this is hydroxylated rapidly to produce β-ecdysone (figure 2.11). It is this latter steroid which is the active moulting hormone. Ecdysteroids initiate moulting by acting on the epidermal cells to cause apolysis (the separation of the old cuticle from the epidermis) and subsequently, formation of the new cuticle and absorption of the old endocuticle. Unfortunately, the mechanism of the early and direct action of ecdysteroids in causing apolysis has been little studied. Most research has concentrated on the role of ecdysteroids in cuticular

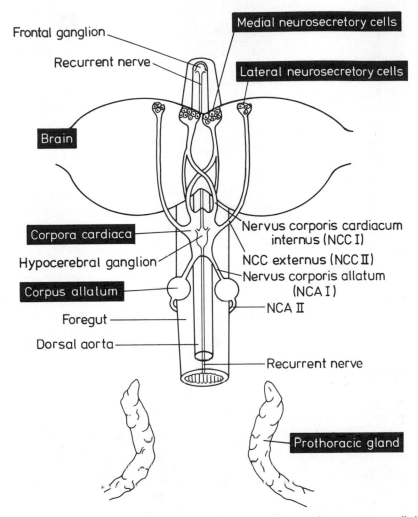

Frontal ganglion

Recurrent nerve

Medial neurosecretory cells

Lateral neurosecretory cells

Brain

Corpora cardiaca

Hypocerebral ganglion

Corpus allatum

Foregut

Dorsal aorta

Nervus corporis cardiacum internus (NCC I)

NCC externus (NCC II)

Nervus corporis allatum (NCA I)

NCA II

Recurrent nerve

Prothoracic gland

Figure 6.1 Diagram of the insect endocrine system. Two groups of neurosecretory cells in each half of the brain send axons to the corpora cardiaca which are in close association with the dorsal aorta. After Highnam, K. C. and Hill, L., in *The Comparative Endocrinology of the Invertebrates* (2nd edition) Edward Arnold, London, 22, 1977.

sclerotization of the blowfly *puparium* which is formed by retention and tanning (= sclerotization) of the last larval cuticle. Tanning involves the cross-linking of cuticular proteins by a quinone derived from *N*-acetyl dopamine (figure 6.2); this stabilization of proteins gives the cuticle its

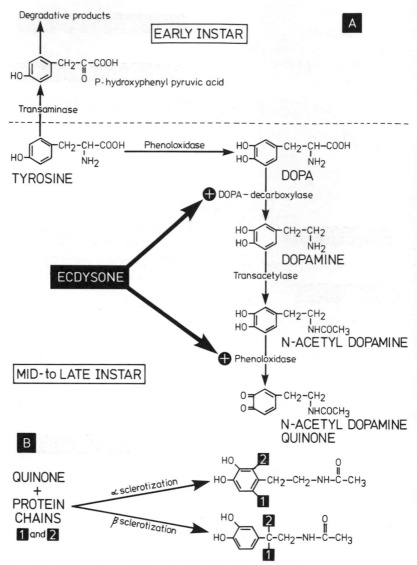

Figure 6.2 A: Tyrosine metabolism in the last larval instar of *Calliphora*. Ecdysone initiates the synthesis of DOPA-decarboxylase, switching tyrosine metabolism from transamination to quinone formation.

B: Possible mechanisms of sclerotin formation by the cross-linking of proteins. β-sclerotization is thought to yield a very hard cuticle whereas α-sclerotization produces a softer, more pliable, tanned cuticle. The two types of sclerotization may, however, proceed simultaneously in the same piece of cuticle.

characteristic hardness and rigidity. The rate-limiting step in the formation of N-acetyl dopamine in the blowfly puparium is the decarboxylation of DOPA (see figure 6.2), and early in the last larval instar, transamination of tyrosine predominates. Later in this instar, ecdysteroids switch tyrosine metabolism towards hydroxylation and decarboxylation; DOPA-decarboxylase activity in the epidermis increases in parallel with the titre of ecdysteroid, and enzyme activity increases in abdomens of ligated larvae (the ligature prevents endogenous release of ecdysteroids) within 10 h of α-ecdysone injection. This response can be prevented by inhibitors of RNA synthesis; mRNA coded for DOPA-decarboxylase is synthesized in response to the ecdysone.

In the blowfly puparium, therefore, ecdysone initiates tanning. During larva-to-larva moults, however, ecdysone causes moulting but does not induce DOPA-decarboxylase activity; the thin cuticle of maggots is not sclerotized. In adult flies, the cuticle is sclerotized shortly after emergence when ecdysteroids are scarcely detectable. Thus, moulting hormone does not always initiate synthesis of DOPA-decarboxylase and, at certain times, enzyme activity increases in the absence of large amounts of ecdysteroid. It is possible that ecdysteroids merely initiate a programme of development appropriate to the state of differentiation of the target tissue (§ 7.7.2). For example, in *Musca autumnalis*, the hardening of the puparium is regulated by ecdysone, but here the hormone controls calcium deposition and sclerotization does not occur.

Bursicon   In many larval and adult insects, tanning of the exocuticle and post-ecdysial deposition of endocuticle are controlled not by ecdysteroids, but by a neurosecretory hormone called *bursicon*. In flies, this hormone is produced by the cerebral neurosecretory cells but released from terminals in the thoracic ganglia; in other insects it is thought to be released by the terminal abdominal ganglia of the ventral nerve cord. Bursicon is a protein of 40 000 molecular weight, is not species specific, and initiates tanning by an action on the haemocytes; it regulates the entry of tyrosine into the blood cells by a cAMP-mediated permeability change allowing its conversion to DOPA by hydroxylation.

Why should insects have two mechanisms for the control of tanning? It is likely that the situation in the blowfly puparium is a special case. The intervention of a second hormone, bursicon, whose release can be determined separately from that of ecdysone, may be a distinct advantage to most insects; species with aquatic stages, and species which develop beneath a substrate or in confined spaces, may require a delay in tanning relative to ecdysis to allow the newly moulted insect to reach the surface before tanning occurs. This will be true especially for the expansion of wings in the adult. Indeed, in the adult blowfly, the signal for bursicon release is only given when this has been achieved.

Crustacea In crustacea most information has come from studies of decapods (especially crabs). Ecdysis is not merely a brief interruption in the life of a crustacean, but a major recurring event which has a profound effect upon its physiology and metabolism. Adult crustacea have been studied most and, unlike our knowledge of insects, little is known of the control of moulting in larvae. Thus, in discussing moulting in arthropods, it is not always possible to compare similar stages in the life history.

In decapods, moulting hormone is released from the Y-organs; when first isolated it was called crustecdysone but it is now known to be identical with β-ecdysone. The overall control of moulting is exercised by the X-organ-sinus gland-neurosecretory complex of the eyestalk (figure

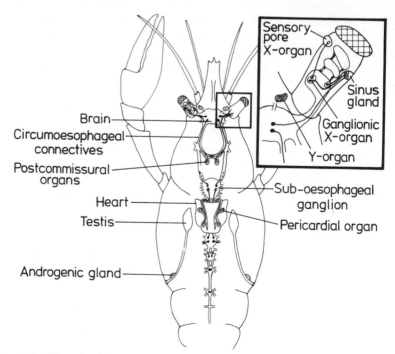

Figure 6.3 The endocrine system of a generalized crustacean. After Gorbman, A. and Bern, H. A., in *A Textbook of Comparative Endocrinology*, John Wiley & Sons, 391, 392, 1962.

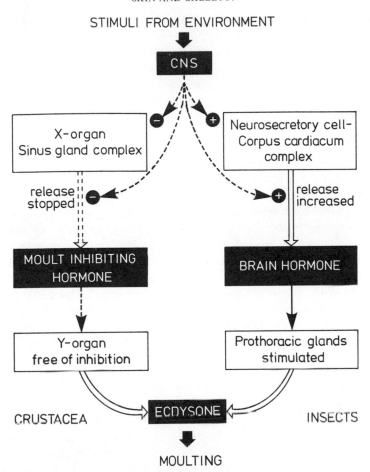

STIMULI FROM ENVIRONMENT

CNS

X-organ
Sinus gland complex

Neurosecretory cell–
Corpus cardiacum
complex

release
stopped

release
increased

MOULT INHIBITING
HORMONE

BRAIN HORMONE

Y-organ
free of inhibition

Prothoracic glands
stimulated

CRUSTACEA   ECDYSONE   INSECTS

MOULTING

Figure 6.4   The hormonal control of moulting in crustaceans and insects.

6.3) which is the source of a moult inhibiting hormone; removal of the eyestalks leads to precocious ecdysis. Thus the control of moulting in insects and crustacea involves a two-step mechanism; neurosecretory hormones control the activity of epithelial endocrine glands and a common steroid hormone affects the target tissues (figure 6.4).

6.1.2   *Vertebrates*
All vertebrates moult, but the detailed nature and endocrine control in different groups varies, not only between classes but also between related

genera. In general, the pituitary and thyroid hormones are implicated as primary controlling agents; the pituitary produces several hormones but TSH, prolactin and ACTH are commonly implicated. Although moulting (= sloughing) in snakes is a familiar occurrence, the complex variations in hormone involvement are especially noticeable in reptiles (and amphibia). We shall, therefore, concentrate our attention on the mammals, where a clearer picture may emerge.

Mammals   By moulting, a mammal can change the colour (see §6.2.2) or insulating properties of the integument. Such moults are usually seasonal and, in general, a spring hair replacement produces a sparse pelage of coarse hairs, through which air easily circulates; in the autumn, a dense pelage of fine hairs is produced which traps warm air and thus increases the insulation properties of the integument. In animals like the deer, however, increased insulation is not dependent on hair density but on enlarged medullary spaces in the guard hairs, e.g. in the roe deer, *Capreolus*, the winter guard hairs are twice the diameter of summer guard hairs. In addition, all mammals have sebaceous glands which coat the skin and hair with a waterproof layer, but large mammals also have apocrine sweat glands over the general body surface which are clearly important in increasing evaporative heat loss. The size and activity of both types of gland vary seasonally and are controlled by hormones—principally androgens in males and possibly progesterone in females.

The environmental factors which initiate moulting also influence seasonal breeding, and there is a close correlation between moulting cycles and gonadal cycles. Thus in the field vole, *Microtus*, the spring moult occurs when the pituitary, gonads, thyroid and adrenal cortex are actively secreting, whereas the autumn moult coincides with regression of these glands. In particular, thyroid hormones initiate hair growth and adreno-cortical hormones encourage loss of mature hairs. Gonadal hormones inhibit hair growth, so that under the influence of increased thyroid, adrenal and gonadal activity in spring, voles grow fewer, coarser hairs— the summer coat. In autumn, lower levels of sex hormones allow more hairs to grow, while mature hairs are retained due to reduced adrenal activity; the hairs produced are finer because thyroid secretion is low and the voles grow a dense pelage of fine hairs—the winter coat.

In other mammals, moulting of the hair may occur more or less continuously and large areas of the body moult synchronously. Man is an exception: each hair follicle undergoes a moult cycle independently of its neighbours. In rats and other small rodents, hair loss and activation of hair follicles is not seasonal but follows a regular pattern governed by intrinsic characteristics of particular areas of skin. By dyeing the hairs of laboratory rats, this cycle is easily observed when new white hairs appear amongst the dyed hairs. The moulting pattern, which is little affected by grafting to other regions, and is therefore largely autonomous, starts on the belly and spreads slowly to the back and head. The effects of hormones on this cycle are consistent with those described for the field vole.

6.2 Hormones and colour change

The integument of most animals contains pigment in the epidermis, dermis or in integumental outgrowths such as scales, hair, feathers etc. The variety of animal colours illustrates the extremely varied chemical composition of the pigments utilized by different animals. However, colours may also result from the physical properties of the skin. In some animals the ability to change colour may be restricted to the sudden exposure of coloured areas, whereas in others the process takes longer and may be complex, involving a number of organs and cellular events which alter the amount of pigment exposed. It is this latter type of colour change with which we shall be concerned. It can occur in two distinct ways. One, called morphological colour change, involves slow long-term changes; the other is physiological colour change which is concerned with rapid short-term changes. Morphological colour changes involve the formation and/or destruction of pigment. Physiological colour change is effected by rapid alterations in the distribution of existing pigments within the epidermis. Both mechanisms are influenced by, and in some animals are under the total control of, hormones.

6.2.1 Physiological colour change

Only a small number of animals are able to change colour rapidly. Amongst the vertebrates the phenomenon is restricted to some poikilotherms, and in the invertebrates is of common occurrence only in cephalopod molluscs and some crustacea. Pigments subject to rapid changes in distribution are found in two types of specialized cells called chromatophores. One type is a thin-walled sac of pigment to which muscle fibres are attached radially; contraction and relaxation of the muscles produces colour changes. This type of chromatophore is found only in the cephalopod molluscs and is under solely nervous control. The other form of chromatophore is present in all other animals showing physiological colour change, with the exception of insects (figure 6.5). The structure of

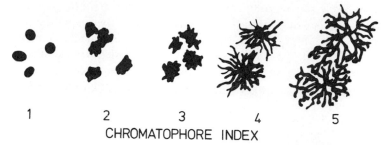

1   2   3   4   5

CHROMATOPHORE INDEX

Figure 6.5 Diagrammatic representation of the Chromatophore Index which is used to make quantitative estimations of dispersion or concentration of pigment.

this latter type of chromatophore is uniformly that of a cell with many dendritic arms branching out from a central core. The pigments are contained in discrete organelles associated with microtubules or other cytoplasmic elements. When the pigment is fully dispersed, it adds colour to the appearance of the animal, but when it is fully concentrated it is not discernible (see figure 6.5). The mechanism by which granules move within the chromatophore is not fully understood, but colchicine and cyto-chalasin B, which interfere with microtubule and microfilament function, inhibit pigment movement. These drugs have other actions in, for example, inhibiting Na^+/K^+-ATPase activity; in Crustacea there is evidence that hormonally induced red pigment dispersion is Ca^{++}-dependent while concentration is Na^+-dependent, so care is required in the interpretation of the action of such drugs. In both crustacea and vertebrates, cAMP is also implicated in the control of pigment movement.

In order to allow comparisons between work from different laboratories and between different species, the degree of pigment dispersion within the chromatophores is often given a value according to the scale given in figure 6.5. This value is known as the Chromatophore (or, in vertebrates, Melanophore) Index, CI (or MI).

Invertebrates   In the decapod crustacea a number of species control their chromatophores hormonally. The X-organ-sinus gland complex in the eyestalks, and the brain-post-commissural organ complex (figure 6.3) produce pigment-dispersing and pigment-aggregating neurosecretory hormones. The chromatophores are numerous and varied, including melanophores, erythrophores, xanthophores and leucophores. They may be unichromatic or polychromatic, with more than one hormone acting simultaneously on the same chromatophore (each hormone acting upon

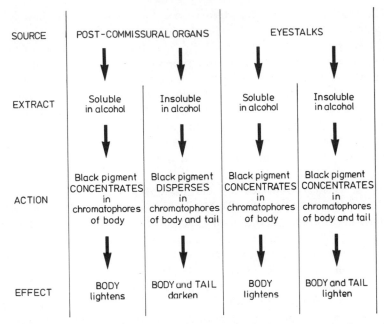

Figure 6.6 Control of dispersion of the black pigment within the chromatophores of the shrimp (*Crangon*). Extraction of the eyestalk or post-commissural organs with alcohol reveals the presence of four different hormones involved. After Highnam, K. C. and Hill, L., in *The Comparative Endocrinology of the Invertebrates* (2nd edition) Edward Arnold, 243, 1977.

different pigment granules). The distribution of a particular pigment is in many instances controlled by antagonistic hormones (figure 6.6); their balance allows intermediate states of pigment dispersion to be maintained. The structures of two of the hormones are known (figure 6.7).

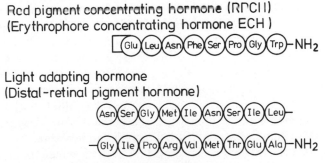

Figure 6.7 Two chromotophorins identified in crustacea.

The primary stimulus for release of colour change hormones is the perception of light by the eyes. The effect of differential illumination of the decapod eye is of prime importance in regulating the release of hormones from the eyestalks and the post-commissural organs. In the sea slater *Ligia*, illumination from the ventral surface which occurs, for example, by reflection from a light background, leads to the release of a melanin-concentrating hormone and the animal pales to tone with the background. If the dorsal or lateral regions of the eye are illuminated, or illuminated more than the ventral region, as would occur on a dark background, a melanin-dispersing hormone is released and the animal darkens.

Vertebrates   In vertebrates the chromatophores commonly contain a black or brown pigment called melanin and these cells are called melanophores; other deposits of melanin which show only long-term changes are held in melanocytes. Other pigments, which are often static, are contained in xanthophores (yellow) and erythrophores (red); some chromatophores contain pteridine platelets, which act as reflectors. In general it is the movement of melanins controlled by hormones, which effects colour changes by altering the amounts of melanin (and other pigments) exposed, or, for the pteridines, the amount of reflected light.

The most important hormone in the regulation of physiological and morphological colour changes in vertebrates is MSH (melanophore/melanocyte stimulating hormone). This peptide is released from the intermediate lobe of the pituitary and has been fully characterized. However, it should be realized that evidence for its existence in lower vertebrates depends on physiological studies and bioassays rather than chemical identification. MSH has been isolated and chemically character-ized only in mammals, which do not exhibit physiological colour change! Indeed, the function of MSH in birds and mammals is uncertain. Its striking structural affinities with ACTH, and β-lipotropin suggest that all of these hormones derive from a single molecule (§2.2.2). We know that several hormones of this family have been selected as physiologically useful in higher vertebrates. Possibly MSH is a redundant molecule, a biochemical vestige retained in these groups. Its survival within the gene pool may have resulted from selection pressure for the parental molecule, rather than from any advantage conferred by MSH itself. Clearly, however, this view could be premature: it is perhaps more likely that MSH in birds and mammals has some function as yet undiscovered.

The control of MSH release is complex. The predominant hypothalamic influence is inhibitory; if the pituitary is removed and reimplanted in the

kidney capsule, for example, or if the nervous connections between the
hypothalamus and the pituitary are cut, MSH is released continuously.
The pathway for communication between the hypothalamus and the
intermediate lobe of the pituitary is by no means clear. In fish and
amphibians this lobe is poorly vascularized but richly innervated by

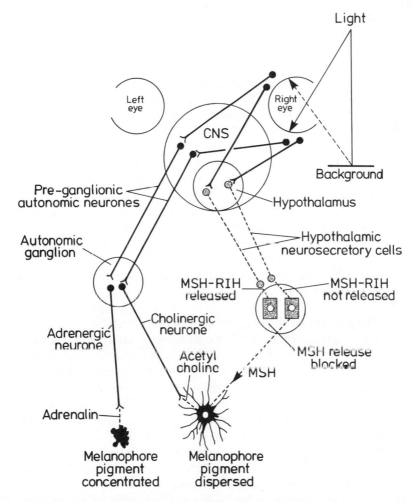

Figure 6.8 Generalized scheme for the control of melanophores in vertebrates. MSH-
RIH = MSH-release-inhibiting hormone. After Scharrer, E. and Scharrer, B., in *Neuroendocrinology*, Columbia University Press, 179, 1963.

hypothalamic aminergic neurons. In higher vertebrates the vascular-
ization is well developed and the innervation reduced. In mammals, there
is evidence for the existence of releasing and release-inhibiting peptides, in
addition to control by aminergic, cholinergic and peptidergic neurones
which terminate in the intermediate lobe. Finally, to complicate matters
further, the pineal gland may also control MSH release. This may be
especially important in photoperiodic control of pigmentation changes
(see § 6.2.2).

Amphibia   Amphibia illustrate the principles of MSH action and the
control of its release most clearly. When placed on a white background,
with overhead illumination, frogs become maximally pale (MI = 1.5); on a
black illuminated background the frog darkens (MI = 4.5). These effects
are due to the differential illumination of the retina (figure 6.8). In a black
tank the frog receives light only on the more basal regions of the retina but
in a white tank light is reflected from all sides and the substratum, so that
all of the retina including the dorsal region is illuminated. Stimulation of
the various regions of the retina elicits different responses from the
hypothalamus (figure 6.8).

  The release of melatonin (see below) from the pineal gland controls the
rhythm of colour change in tadpoles but the hormone is not involved in
skin lightening in adults; in adults pallor results solely from the decline in
MSH titre. Amphibian chromatophores are not innervated but in some
reptiles and fish, nerves control melanin aggregation while hormones
cause pigment dispersal.

6.2.2   *Morphological colour change*

Hormonal control over the production and destruction of integumentary
pigments is of limited occurrence in invertebrates, and has been described
only in insects. In locusts, neurosecretory hormones promote deposition of
black pigment in response to high population densities and/or low
temperature and high relative humidity. Juvenile hormone (figure 2.12)
controls the deposition of a green pigment in the blood and cuticle of
solitary phase locusts, and the yellow colour of sexually mature locusts. In
other insects such as the tobacco hornworm moth, *Manduca*, the ability of
juvenile hormone to influence the formation of characteristic pigments in
the cuticle forms the basis of a sensitive bioassay.

  In vertebrates the role of hormones in the control of morphological
changes in integumentary colours is well established. The sex steroid
hormones, MSH, LH, melatonin and ACTH may be all involved but their

detailed roles are less clear than in the hormonal control of physiological colour change. Melanin is the pigment affected most often but other pigments are involved in animals which show marked sexual dimorphism, seasonal colour changes, or changes associated with sexual cycles. In finches, for example, the sexually mature male is brightly coloured with red or orange feathers and the growth of this plumage is prevented by castration; the feathers which develop are the dull-coloured female type. It is likely that the synthesis of the brightly coloured pigments is controlled by androgens.

Marked colour changes are often seen during the seasonal changes in pelage exhibited by mammals such as hares, deer and weasels. Weasels, for example, change their coat from brown to white with the onset of winter. In the laboratory, they maintain their brown pelage when kept in an artificial photoperiod of 12 h light/12 h dark. Hypophysectomy causes the production of a white pelage, whereas if the removed pituitary is implanted under the kidney capsule, brown hairs develop at the next moult— presumably due to uncontrolled release of MSH from the denervated pituitary. Hair colour in hypophysectomized weasels is unaffected by photoperiod. When hair growth is initiated locally in hypophysectomized weasels, by plucking out hairs, the new hairs which grow are white unless the animal is treated with MSH, when brown hairs develop at the site of plucking (surrounded by unaffected white hairs). Clearly the effect of MSH on hair colour requires activation of the hair follicles—by plucking in this case.

It is likely that the normal seasonal changes of coat are subject to photoperiodic control via the endocrine system. We have seen that the moult cycle appears to be linked with cycles of activity in the gonads, adrenal, and thyroid glands (§ 6.1.2), as well as being influenced by MSH in those animals with a seasonal colour-change. There is increasing evidence that the pineal gland mediates photoperiodic control over sexual cycles in mammals and birds. The pineal is thought to synthesize melatonin (from 5-hydroxytryptamine) under the influence of a biological clock situated in the hypothalamus; a circadian rhythm of melatonin production results. In many vertebrates, melatonin inhibits growth of the gonads, and subcutaneous implantation of a melatonin-beeswax mixture (which allows slow and prolonged release of the melatonin) in male weasels causes them to become reproductively quiescent and grow a white coat instead of the normal brown spring coat. It is uncertain whether this is a direct effect of melatonin on MSH release or an indirect effect via the gonad.

6.3   Hormones and the skeleton

It is often difficult to identify effects of hormones specifically upon the skeletal system. In general, hormones which regulate growth and/or moulting affect the growth of the skeleton. Growth of the mollusc shell is intimately concerned with calcium metabolism and in Lymnaea is controlled by the light-green neurosecretory cells of the cerebral ganglia (figure 7.17). Similarly, in crustaceans, calcium is an essential component of the exoskeleton and its metabolism is regulated during the moult. In vertebrates, however, there is a precise and specific hormonal control of calcium metabolism which is worthy of separate consideration.

6.3.1   *Hormones and calcium metabolism in mammals*

Precise regulation of calcium in blood and other body fluids is essential because ionic calcium forms not only a major component of the endo-skeleton but also has important metabolic effects on membrane per-meability, enzyme activity, muscle contraction and neural transmission etc. Calcium levels are influenced by three major centres (figure 6.9)—the small intestine, the kidney and the skeleton. The flux of Ca^{++} between these organs, the body fluids and the intestine is controlled by three hormones—calcitonin, parathyroid hormone (parathormone, PTH), and a hormonal derivative of vitamin D called 1,25-dihydroxycholecalciferol (1,25-DHCC).

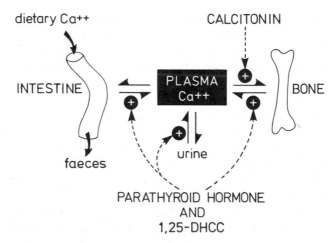

Figure 6.9   The regulation of blood calcium in birds and mammals. After Copp, D. H. (1969) *J. Endocr.*, **43**, 137–161.

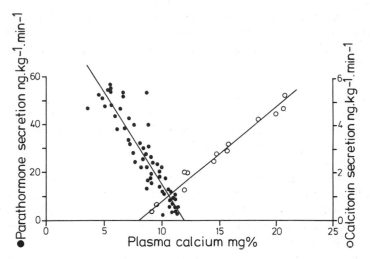

Figure 6.10 Calcium feedback control of parathormone and calcitonin secretion in mammals. After Copp, D. H. (1969) *J. Endocr.*, **43**, 137–161.

Calcitonin is released from the "C" cells of the mammalian thyroid, and induces hypocalcaemia by inhibiting osteolysis (bone demineralization). There is a linear relationship between its release into the blood and increased circulatory levels of Ca^{++} (figure 6.10).

The secretion of PTH is regulated directly by the blood calcium level. A sensitive feedback mechanism operates such that a decline in blood calcium elicits the synthesis and release of PTH; the relationship is a linear one (figure 6.10). PTH stimulates osteolysis, releasing calcium and phosphate from bone, and increases phosphate excretion in the urine. The net effect being a return of blood calcium to normal. Another important effect of PTH is to stimulate the production of 1,25-DHCC.

Vitamin D is a steroid and, as is indicated by its name, is a dietary requirement. It can also be formed in the skin as vitamin D_3, cholecalciferol, from 7-dehydrocholesterol by the action of ultra-violet light. Cholecalciferol is oxidized first in the liver and again in the kidneys to produce the active hormone, 1,25-DHCC. Its production is stimulated by low levels of calcium and phosphate, whereas high plasma levels of these ions lead to the formation of a relatively inactive metabolite of vitamin D_3. The intake of dietary Ca^{++} and phosphate across the intestinal wall is controlled by 1,25-DHCC which regulates the synthesis in the gut and bone cells of a protein which carries Ca^{++} into the blood. The balance of

Ca^{++} and phosphate levels in the bone is regulated therefore by the interactions of these three hormones. PTH and 1,25-DHCC act synergistically in increasing osteolysis, while calcitonin directly opposes this effect.

6.3.2 *Calcium regulation in lower vertebrates*

In lower vertebrates, calcium regulation is often closely associated with osmoregulatory phenomena, especially in aquatic forms; in soft fresh water they face the problem of calcium loss but marine forms must limit its entry and actively excrete any excess.

The role of the parathyroid glands in calcium regulation in birds, reptiles, anuran amphibia and higher urodeles, is probably similar to that in mammals. Parathyroid glands are, however, absent in fishes; in these and lower urodeles, prolactin may have an important hypercalcaemic role.

The ultimobranchial bodies, homologues of the C cells of the mammalian thyroid, are present in all non-mammalian jawed vertebrates and produce calcitonins. There seems little doubt that these are important in calcium regulation in lower vertebrates but injected calcitonin does not exert consistent hypocalcaemic responses in many non-mammalian vertebrates. However, its chronic administration in young birds and turtles increases calcium deposition in bone, and in young trout aids survival in calcium deficient media.

Teleosts possess unique glandular structures, the corpuscles of Stannius, which are closely associated with the kidneys. When fish are kept in calcium rich media, removal of these corpuscles results in hypercalcaemia which can be corrected by injections of extracts of the corpuscles. These extracts contain a low molecular weight glycopeptide which restricts calcium entry by inhibiting its active transport across the gills.

The corpuscles of Stannius also contain a renin-like material which, when incubated with blood plasma, releases an angiotensin with marked hypocalcaemic activity: kidney renin produces an angiotensin which is less active in this respect. It is thought that the renin-like material and glycopeptide are separate molecules. Clearly, the physiological role of the corpuscles of Stannius requires further study.

CHAPTER SEVEN

REPRODUCTION AND MORPHOGENESIS

IN 1849 BERTHOLD PERFORMED WHAT WAS TO BECOME AN ARCHETYPAL ENDOCRINE experiment. He transplanted a testis from a sexually mature cockerel into a castrate male (capon) and subsequently observed the restoration of comb growth in the recipient bird. Pezard, in 1911, showed that a saline extract of cockerel testis could substitute for such a transplant. These simple experiments involving *ablation* followed by *replacement* were to have significance far beyond the study of avian reproduction: they laid the foundation of present day endocrinology.

With this historical perspective, the aims of this chapter may be stated. It is not our intention to present a comparative account of reproductive endocrinology: to do so is clearly outside the scope and general rationale of this book. Our approach will be selective, using as a framework information now available to describe endocrine mechanisms which have general significance beyond that relating solely to reproductive function.

7.1   The hypothalamo-pituitary-gonadal axis

As vertebrates evolved, the hypothalamus came to occupy a central role in the control of reproduction. The mammalian hypothalamus, in particular, has been shown to function as a remarkable integration centre, capable of processing numerous and diverse informational inputs; appropriate hormonal responses are directed via the anterior and posterior pituitary (figure 7.1).

Hormonal feedback which influences hypothalamic output of releasing factors is derived from three sources (see also § 2.3):

113

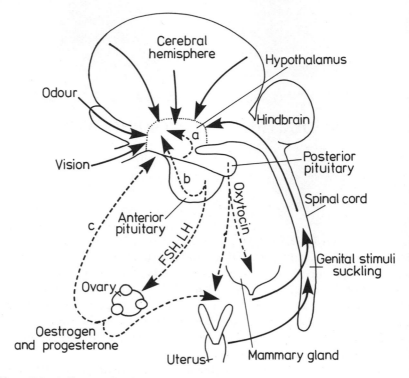

Figure 7.1 A diagram showing the various nervous inputs (solid arrows) and hormonal influences (broken arrows) impinging on the hypothalamus. Some of the main target organs of the reproductive hormones from the pituitary are shown. Note the three hormonal feedbacks: ultra-short loop (*a*) from the hypothalamus itself, short loop (*b*) from the anterior pituitary, and long loop (*c*) from the ovary. After Cross, B. A., in *Reproduction in Mammals*, Vol. 3 (C. R. Austin and R. V. Short, eds.) C.U.P., 34, Cambridge, 1972.

(i) *ultra-short loop*, in which the rate of release of hypothalamic neurosecretion negatively modulates itself directly;

(ii) *short loop*, again negative, from anterior pituitary hormones, synthesized and released in response to hypothalamic releasing hormones;

(iii) *long loop*, from gonadal steroid hormones, synthesized and released in response to gonadotropic stimulation.

This latter feedback is worth examining in further detail (figure 7.2). The modulation of hypothalamic discharge of gonadotropin releasing hormone (Gn-RH, figure 7.3) by gonadal steroids is usually negative in character. For example, injection of testosterone lowers circulating luteinizing hormone (LH), which is released in response to Gn-RH;

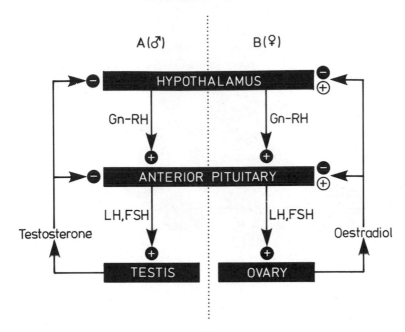

Figure 7.2 Feedback between the gonads and the hypothalamus/anterior pituitary in sexually mature male (A) and female (B) mammals. In the male the feedback is always negative; in the female, oestradiol usually modulates gonadotropin release negatively, but a positive feedback occurs prior to ovulation in each oestrous cycle.

conversely, gonadotropins are elevated after castration. While this type of relationship is invariably seen in male mammals, it is not always so in females: rising levels of oestradiol, produced by maturing Graafian follicles (figure 7.4) are responsible for triggering a massive release of LH— the "LH surge"—and hence ovulation. Thus positive feedback is an important component of ovarian cyclicity (see also §7.4.1). This difference in functional capability between the male and female hypothalamus is an interesting example of sexual differentiation, and we now know that it is programmed very early in life—either before birth, or in the neonatal

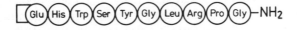

Figure 7.3   Gonadotropin releasing hormone (Gn-RH).

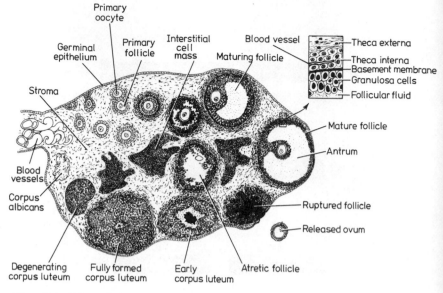

Figure 7.4   Schematic diagram of a mammalian ovary, showing the sequence of events in the origin, growth, and rupture of the Graafian follicle, and the formation and regression of the corpus luteum. After Gorbman, A. and Bern, H. A., in *A Textbook of Comparative Endocrinology*, John Wiley & Sons, 253, New York, 1962.

period. Under the influence of fetal testicular steroids, the potential for the positive feedback component (figure 7.2B) is lost, and a male-type hypothalamus/pituitary results. A similar result can be achieved in genotypically female mammals by a single injection of testosterone during the critical period of early life. Subsequent development is normal except that after puberty the regular pattern of ovarian cyclicity never develops, and the individual is sterile.

The hypothalamus also receives nervous input from a variety of sources (figure 7.1). Vision and olfaction are important neural routes involved in coordinating reproductive function via the hypothalamus. A change in photoperiod (i.e. shortening or increasing day length) is the environmental cue perceived by many species of mammal and bird which triggers increased hypothalamic release of Gn-RH and hence elevated gonado-tropin output, renewed gonadal activity and the onset of a "breeding season" (see also § 7.4.2). For example, sheep mate in the autumn because their annual sexual maturation is synchronized by the hypothalamic response to decreasing day length. Olfaction also plays a role in several aspects of reproductive behaviour in mammals: in many species the male will only initiate sexual activity with a female in oestrus (§ 7.4.1), after detecting the characteristic odour of a pheromonal secretion produced in the female reproductive tract at this time. Similarly male pheromones, often deposited in the urine, can coordinate female sexual behaviour: a few drops of urine from a sexually mature male mouse is often sufficient, when introduced into a cage of anoestrous female mice, to stimulate renewed ovarian activity and the return of synchronized oestrous cycles (the "Whitten effect").

The hypothalamus responds also to neural inputs coming via the spinal cord (figure 7.1). If the response provoked is hormonal, the sequence can be described as a *neuro-endocrine reflex*; the afferent arc is nervous, the efferent arc is hormonal. There are numerous examples of such reflexes in mammalian reproductive physiology. In lactating females, oxytocin (synthesized in cell bodies of the paraventricular nucleus of the hypothalamus (figure 1.1) is released from the posterior pituitary as an acute response to stimulation of the nipple during suckling (the "milk-ejection reflex"). Uterine and cervical distension also trigger oxytocin release during parturition (§ 7.5), and orgasm in the human female is also associated with oxytocin release. Hormonal output from the anterior pituitary can also be modulated by neuro-endocrine reflexes: an ovulatory surge of LH is released in response to cervical stimulation (from copulation, or direct artificial means) in those female mammals which are "induced ovulators", such as the rabbit, cat, ferret and mink. The duration of this reflex is relatively long and in the rabbit, for example, ovulation occurs about 12 hours after mating.

As a final example of hypothalamic response to neural input, the modulating influence, at least in humans, of higher brain centres can be mentioned. A glance through the "agony" columns of many women's magazines will often provide evidence suggestive of such pathways. Reproductive function in the human female can be disturbed by a variety of emotional traumas, producing symptoms ranging from irregular or absent menses, to pseudopregnancy. Nor is the human male exempt from similar influences; beard growth, which is androgen- and hence LH- and Gn-RH-dependent, increases in anticipation of female company, following a period of sexual abstinence.

In summary, the hypothalamus can be described as having a central role in the coordination of reproductive processes. It has a similar integrative function in many other endocrine systems (such as those involved in growth, or responses to stress, and cold acclimation). Indeed the hypo-

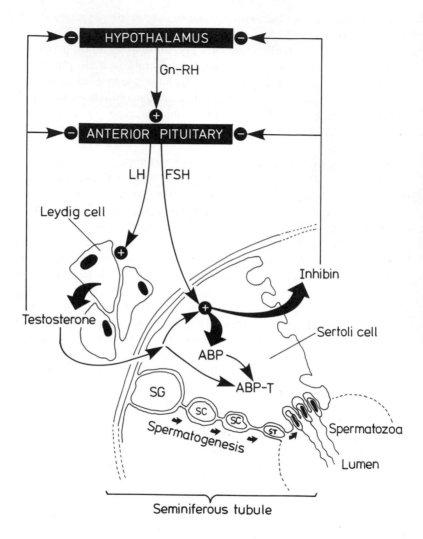

Figure 7.5 Diagram showing the functional dichotomy of mammalian testis. Leydig cells, the target tissue for LH, are sites of hormone (testosterone) biosynthesis. Within the seminiferous tubules Sertoli cells support the germ cells. The stages of spermatogenesis are indicated, starting (peripherally) with spermatogonia (SG), primary and secondary spermatocytes (SC) and spermatids (ST). Two characteristic products of Sertoli cells are shown: *androgen-binding protein* (ABP) binds testosterone, and *inhibin* (a small peptide) probably negatively modulates FSH release.

thalamus controls a host of physiological homeostatic mechanisms; a truly remarkable capability in an organ which, in the human, is itself only about 0.004 % of the weight of the whole brain.

7.2 Testicular function

Whilst the principal activity of the testis is the production of spermatozoa, the organ also has an important endocrinological function in the biosynthesis and release of steroid hormones—*androgens*. Testicular structure reflects this functional dichotomy (figure 7.5): spermatogenesis is confined to the long, tightly convoluted, seminiferous tubules which constitute about 95 % of the testis mass, whereas steroidogenesis is initiated in the interstitial (or Leydig) cells. The intertubular region is richly perfused by blood capillaries, in contrast to the seminiferous tubules which are avascular, being isolated behind the "blood-testis" barrier (figure 7.5).

Testosterone is the major androgenic hormone secreted by the Leydig

Table 7.1 The biochemical effects of androgens on target organs of male animals (higher vertebrates).

Organ	Species	Developmental Period	Effect
External genitalia (e.g. penis)	All	Embryonic	Sexual differentiation
Accessory sex glands (e.g. prostate)	All	Pubertal	Rapid growth and stimulation of secretions
Testis	All	Pubertal	Spermatogenesis
Brain	Most	Fetal or neonatal	Sexual differentiation
Brain	All	Adult	Libido
Liver	Most	Embryonic	Haemoglobin synthesis
Blastoderm	Birds only	Embryonic	Haemoglobin synthesis
Liver	Most	Neonatal	Synthesis of enzymes
Kidney	Mouse	Adult	Enzyme synthesis and cellular hypertrophy
Salivary gland	Pig	Adult	Pheromone production
Muscle	Most	Pubertal	Slow growth (anabolic effect)
Hair follicles in specific areas	Most	Pubertal	Hair growth
Sebaceous glands	Most	Pubertal	Sebaceous secretion
Bone marrow	Most	Adult	RNA and protein synthesis
Vocal cords	Most	Pubertal	Thickening of cords

cells of most adult vertebrates, and its biosynthesis is controlled by the stimulatory action of LH. As we have said, testosterone modulates the release of LH by depressing hypothalamic output of Gn-RH (figure 7.3), but testosterone-induced desensitization of the anterior pituitary's responsiveness to the releasing hormone may also be involved in this feedback relationship (figure 7.5). FSH is not involved in controlling steroidogenic activity in Leydig cells, nor are any of the components of the seminiferous tubules capable of *de novo* synthesis of steroids.

Testosterone is an excellent example of a hormone which has numerous different targets. The responses embody a wide spectrum of physiological and behavioural changes ranging from the exotic plumage and courtship displays of many male birds to the more mundane propensity of a dog to cock his leg. Some idea of the wide range of androgenic effects is conveyed in table 7.1 but this list is by no means comprehensive.

Another characteristic of testosterone that has a general endocrinological significance is its role as a prohormone (§3.4.2). Testosterone is converted in some target tissues to a "superactive" metabolite. This was first recognized in connection with the peripheral production of 5-α-dihydrotestosterone, but there is growing evidence that other biologically active metabolites exist. These vary depending on the target system involved (figure 7.6) and in at least one instance, the resulting "active" hormone is not a recognized androgen, but, paradoxically, oestradiol. The sexual differentiation of the hypothalamic feedback potentiality (figure 7.2) is programmed after exposure to androgens released from the fetal testis which become aromatized to oestradiol (figure 7.6) within the hypothalamus.

The hormonal control of spermatogenesis is not as clearly understood as that relating to steroid hormone biosynthesis in the testis. After hypophysectomy the weight of the testis rapidly declines as both spermatogenesis and steroidogenesis cease. If LH replacement is begun immediately after hypophysectomy of the adult male rat, testicular functions are maintained; administration of testosterone in relatively large amounts can replace LH in this situation. The initiation of spermatogenesis, as opposed to its maintenance, requires FSH. Recent research suggests that the major and perhaps only action of LH in spermatogenesis is indirect, exerted by testosterone produced in the Leydig cells (figure 7.5). Neither Sertoli nor germ cells possess LH-binding activity. The testis itself is therefore an important target for testosterone. The Sertoli cells' response involves increased secretory activity including the biosynthesis of a unique androgen-binding protein (ABP). FSH, which does have receptors on

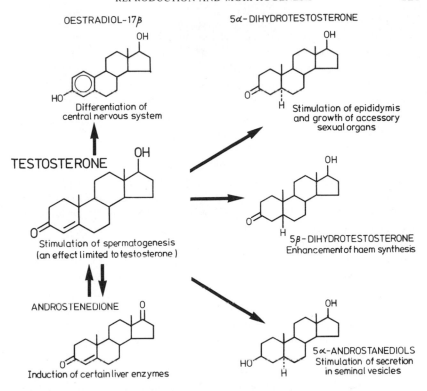

Figure 7.6 The structure of testosterone and its biologically active metabolites, with an indication of their functions. From Mainwaring, W. I. P., in *Reproduction in Mammals*, Vol. 7 (C. R. Austin and R. V. Short, eds.) C.U.P., 122, Cambridge, 1979.

Sertoli (but not Leydig) cells, also stimulates ABP formation and in addition, that of a peptide called "inhibin". Inhibin is probably responsible for the selective feedback control of FSH output from the anterior pituitary (figure 7.5). How Sertoli cells influence spermatogenesis is not yet known. Their general function may be to provide a supportive environment for the maturational divisions of the developing germ cells within the blood-testis barrier. Testosterone is implicated in the regulation of some of these processes. By binding testosterone avidly, ABP is responsible for creating a localized high concentration of this steroid within the seminiferous tubule, which might be necessary for spermatogenesis or sperm maturation to proceed.

7.3   The ovary

The ovary, like the testis, is concerned with both gamete and hormone production. However, a striking difference between the gonads is seen when spermatogenesis and oogenesis are compared. Once puberty is passed spermatogenesis is a continuous process, although it may often be seasonally restricted (§ 7.4.2). In contrast, the mitotic stages of oogenesis in female mammals are usually complete before birth, providing the ovary with a limited store of primary oocytes (figure 7.4) to serve the reproductive lifespan. The human ovary, in the newborn, contains about 2 million of these germ cells, of which about 300 000 will persist until puberty. Throughout her reproductive years a woman might ovulate about 400 oocytes—and yet by the time the menopause is reached the ovarian store is virtually empty. Clearly the fate of most oocytes (and indeed spermatozoa) is not fertilization.

Oocyte development up to the point of ovulation takes place within ovarian (Graafian) follicles, and is shown schematically in figure 7.4. Virtually all the changes seen are those involving growth, differentiation and maturation of the follicles. Further maturation of the oocyte—the resumption of meiosis—begins just prior to ovulation and usually is not completed until after sperm penetration.

The recruitment of ovarian follicles, their maturation and eventual fate is controlled hormonally. The manner in which this is achieved has fascinated generations of reproductive endocrinologists. Although much remains to be discovered the picture that emerges is one of extraordinary complex interrelationships between cells, and many of the mechanisms that have been recently elucidated may have a wide relevance in other areas of endocrine function.

In common with other protein hormones, FSH, LH, and prolactin interact with their targets by binding to specific receptors present on cell surfaces (although subsequent involvement of the hormone within the cell now appears probable; see § 4.1.10). The progressive growth of an ovarian follicle seems to be associated largely with changes in its receptor population, which in turn allow the follicle to respond to circulating hormones and develop new functional capabilities as maturation proceeds.

The early stages of follicle growth involve FSH; primary follicles do not contain LH receptors, but their granulosa cells (figure 7.4 above) possess FSH receptors. FSH probably is responsible for recruiting follicles from their ovarian "pool" and stimulates their growth. Only when the follicle has reached a "medium" size, do receptors for another gonadotropin, LH, develop within it. At this stage the thecal layers have developed around the basement membrane of the follicle, and the LH receptors seem to be exclusively located on these cells. Thecal cells can synthesize steroids, and in response to LH they produce androgens. Granulosal cells at this stage appear to have poor steroidogenic competence; while they can convert cholesterol to progesterone, the further metabolism of this steroid is limited, and in particular the final reactions in the pathway to oestrogen biosynthesis (figure 2.9) are deficient. Maturation of the granulosa cells is promoted by FSH under whose influence they divide mitotically, proliferating around the "lining" of the follicle; their increased secretory activity is reflected in the growing volume of follicular fluid, in which the still quiescent oocyte is bathed. One important maturational effect of FSH on granulosal cells at this time is the induction of an enzyme system within them which enables the synthesis of oestradiol from androgens (the "aromatizing" reaction). Thus levels of oestrogens rise within the follicle. It seems likely that some, if not all, of the steroid precursor for oestrogen biosynthesis is "imported" from the androgen secretion of the thecal cells surrounding the follicle (figure 7.7). Oestrogens are potent mitogens, and stimulate the further proliferation of granulosal tissue; they also potentiate FSH actions, which in turn promotes yet more oestrogen formation by a local positive feedback. Follicle size increases dramatically during the period leading up to ovulation. The final crucial maturational effect of FSH which is also potentiated by oestrogen is the induction of receptors for LH on the granulosa cells. These permit the ovulatory actions of LH to be exerted on "pre-ovulatory" follicles after the LH surge arrives (§ 7.4.1); there is little further involvement of FSH in the ovulatory mechanism. LH causes the granulosal cells to *luteinize*, i.e. the cells undergo ultrastructural changes reflecting their transformation into active steroid secreting cells (see figure 2.3) capable of producing progesterone in large amounts. The oocyte at this stage resumes meiosis. LH, like FSH before it, has maturational effects on the granulosa cell receptor population but in this case it is to *reduce* the number of receptors for FSH and LH on the cells' plasma membranes.

After expulsion of the ovum the ruptured follicle(s) becomes the corpus luteum, secreting the steroid hormone largely responsible for the mainten-ance of early pregnancy—progesterone. This steroidogenic function of the corpus luteum requires low levels of LH to sustain it (a "luteotropic" influence). The polypeptide hormone prolactin contributes luteotropic support, partly by inducing and maintaining LH receptors on the corpus luteum.

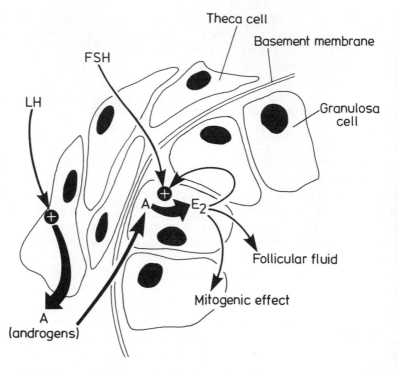

Figure 7.7 Diagram showing cooperation between thecal and granulosal cells during Graafian follicle maturation. Thecal production of androgens (A) provides granulosal cells with steroid precursor for oestrogen (E_2) biosynthesis: the necessary "aromatizing" enzyme is induced by FSH—an effect which is potentiated by oestrogens (i.e. a local positive feedback).

The scenario described above shows several features of general endocrinological importance. The development of a Graafian follicle is characterized by successive changes in its complement of hormone receptors. It is now convincingly clear that hormones regulate the appearance and/or disappearance of hormone receptors in granulosa cells at specific stages of follicular growth. Clearly, regulation of its hormone receptors can crucially affect a cell's function: a response to a hormonal stimulus can be initiated (or terminated) by changing the number of cell receptors present—*even when circulating levels of the hormone remain constant.* This sort of hormone/receptor coordination can be broadly categorized as:

(i)   autoregulation—where a hormone affects the content of its own receptors in target cells (e.g. FSH promotes FSH receptors; LH diminishes LH receptors)

(ii)   heteroregulation—where a hormone affects the levels of receptors for another hormone (e.g. FSH, and prolactin induce LH receptors).

The phenomenon whereby a hormone causes a negative (or "down") regulation of its own receptors, as is the case for LH, is now recognized as a phenomenon which may be common to several hormones and perhaps certain drugs (see §4.1.2). For example, elevated levels of insulin cause a decrease in insulin receptors in target tissues and hence diminishing responsiveness ("desensitization"). The time interval for such events to occur is relatively long (at least 6 hours, often up to 24 hours) and the mechanism involved is unknown. It is not caused by a progressive increase in occupancy of receptors, and is probably too slow to be an allosteric alteration of receptor structure. Cell receptors are not permanent features of a cell's architecture. They are formed, have a short functional life, and are subsequently degraded: the biological half-life of a receptor is short— as indeed is the case with most hormone molecules themselves. "Down regulation" of a receptor population could result from either a decrease in the rate of receptor synthesis, or increase in the rate of its breakdown.

Finally, it seems quite plausible that very localized regulatory mechanisms and inter-cell cooperation such as those which are now recognized in follicle development, will also be found in other endocrine systems.

7.4   Reproductive cyclicity

Many features of reproductive physiology have an apparent cyclicity— some episodic event that recurs in a set pattern. Two such cyclical phenomena are discussed below.

7.4.1   Ovarian cycles

Ovulation is an event that recurs at regular intervals during the reproductive period of a sexually mature female. The most overt sign of such ovarian cyclicity in many mammals is an often stereotyped behaviour pattern during which the sexual attention of mature males is tolerated or even actively solicited. Such recurring periods of female receptivity are termed *oestrus* (= heat), and the cycles in which they occur, *oestrous cycles*. The basis of ovarian cycles is largely endocrine, and investigation of hormone levels as they fluctuate throughout an oestrous cycle has revealed a fascinating pattern of communication between the various components of the reproductive system.

It is likely that there is considerable variation in detail between the oestrous cycles of different mammals but relatively few species have been

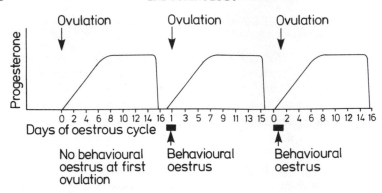

Figure 7.8   The sheep oestrous cycle, showing how the first ovulation of the breeding season is unaccompanied by oestrus. The corpus luteum is active (secreting progesterone) for most of each cycle; after its abrupt demise the next cycle starts and ovulation occurs within a short time. After Short, R. V., in *Reproduction in Mammals*, Vol. 3 (C. R. Austin and R. V. Short, eds.) C.U.P., 54, Cambridge, 1972.

investigated in depth. In recent years studies on sheep have furnished much information about the underlying endocrinology of oestrous cycles (and pregnancy—see § 7.5).

Some of the salient features of sheep oestrous cycles are shown in figure 7.8. Infertile cycles are 16 days in duration, and it is usual to designate the first day on which oestrous behaviour occurs as day 0. Oestrus lasts for about a day, and about 24 hours after its onset ovulation occurs. The corpus luteum then formed begins secreting progesterone, reaching its maximal level of output by day 7. Luteal secretion is sustained at this rate until day 15, at which point *luteolysis*—the functional demise of the corpus luteum—occurs abruptly. As we shall see, this luteal "death" is not from senility, but is better described as "murder". Within 2 days the cycle has ended, another follicle has matured, the next oestrus and ovulation have arrived.

This type of oestrous cycle, similar to that of other large domestic species such as the cow and pig, is one dominated by the corpus luteum: the recruitment and maturation of a new follicle occupies only a small fraction of the cycle duration. Furthermore, if a corpus luteum is destroyed prematurely (e.g. by surgical removal), the time of the next oestrus is advanced. Clearly, in the sheep, the lifespan of the corpus luteum is an important determinant of ovarian cyclicity.

The most significant clue as to the identity of the "murderer" of the corpus luteum comes from experiments involving removal of the uterus—

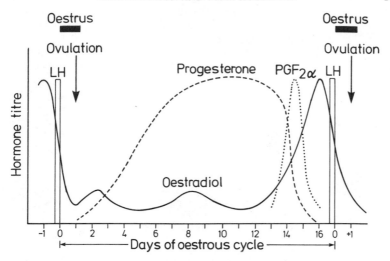

Figure 7.9   The sequence of hormonal events during the sheep oestrous cycle. After Greep, R. O., in *Physiology Series One*, Vol. 8 (R. O. Greep, ed.) Butterworth and Co., 72, London, 1974.

hysterectomy. When this is performed in sheep, the corpus luteum persists for about 165 days. These experiments, and earlier studies in different species, suggest that the uterus produces a "lytic" agent, capable of terminating corpus luteum function, which was given the name *luteolysin*: we now know it to be a prostaglandin designated $PGF_2\alpha$.

The pivotal role of $PGF_2\alpha$ in the control of the sheep oestrous cycle is indicated in figure 7.9. The simplified sequence of hormonal events is as follows, taking day 8 as a convenient starting point. The uterine endometrium is stimulated to synthesize $PGF_2\alpha$ by progesterone from the corpus luteum: in this way the corpus luteum programmes its own destruction. Progesterone also prevents the hypothalamo-pituitary system releasing ovulatory surges of LH, which might occur in response to oestradiol produced during waves of follicle development. The rising level of oestradiol originates in the follicle destined to ovulate in the next cycle, and provokes an increase in endometrial $PGF_2\alpha$ synthesis and release. $PGF_2\alpha$ rapidly terminates luteal secretion, and progesterone levels fall. Rising oestradiol triggers the "LH surge", and ovulation follows. Oestrous behaviour has meanwhile returned, being a response in the sheep to rising oestrogen levels preceded by a decline in progesterone.

Prostaglandin $F_2\alpha$ has been shown to be luteolytic in many mammals.

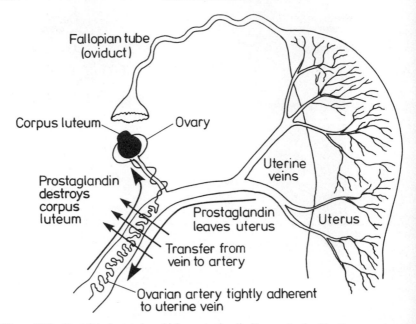

Figure 7.10   Postulated route by which prostaglandin $F_2\alpha$ synthesized by the progesterone-primed uterus is able to enter the ovarian artery and cause corpus luteum regression (luteolysis) in the sheep. From Short, R. V., in *Reproduction in Mammals*, Vol. 3 (C. R. Austin and R. V. Short, eds.) C.U.P., 57, Cambridge, 1972.

In the sheep its route of transfer from the uterus to the ovary (figure 7.10) involves a curious "short-circuit", allowing relatively large amounts of $PGF_2\alpha$ to be transferred directly from the uterine vein to ovarian artery, and thus escape degration in the general circulation. The biochemical mechanism of $PGF_2\alpha$-induced luteolysis is not yet understood. "Functional luteolysis" (i.e. the reduction in luteal progesterone secretion) has a rapid onset, and is well advanced before the appearance of any morphological changes ("structural luteolysis") characteristic of regressing corpora lutea. The current working hypothesis is that $PGF_2\alpha$ interferes with LH-adenylate cyclase interactions, thus rapidly depriving luteal cells of gonadotropic support for steroidogenesis. The initial effect on adenylate cyclase, which is discernible within minutes, is followed several hours later by an irreversible reduction in the number of LH receptors on luteal cells, and the gradual onset of structural luteolysis.

The corpus luteum in the human and other primates is probably not regulated in this way. Hysterectomy does not usually affect human ovarian function, and administration of exogenous $PGF_2\alpha$ produces only a transient decrease in plasma progesterone. Nevertheless receptors for $PGF_2\alpha$ have been demonstrated in the human corpus luteum, and this tissue is capable of synthesizing $PGF_2\alpha$ *in vitro*. Perhaps $PGF_2\alpha$ is produced locally to terminate luteal function: certainly prostaglandins are known to function in very localized regulatory mechanisms elsewhere (see § 4.1.8).

7.4.2 *Seasonal cycles*

After sexual maturity, gonadal function in most mammals and in many other vertebrates is restricted to a specific "breeding" season. The changes that take place in the hypothalamo-pituitary-gonadal system during such annual cycles probably are similar to those that precede puberty. Recent studies on the reactivation of testicular activity in the Soay ram provide a good illustration of the endocrine basis of seasonal sexual cycles. This

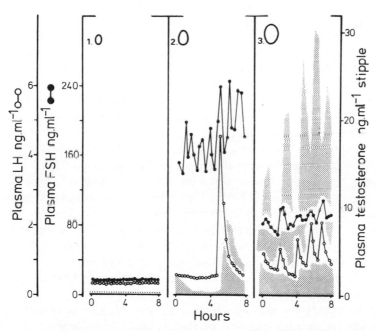

Figure 7.11   Changes in the titres of LH, FSH and testosterone in the blood plasma of one adult Soay ram sampled at 20 min intervals for 8 h on three occasions during the seasonal sexual cycle. 1, testes fully regressed; 2, testes redeveloping; 3, testes fully enlarged, during the mating season. From Lincoln, G. A. (1979) *Brit. Med. Bull.*, **35**(2), 167–172.

work is also of general interest, in that it provides some insight into the mechanism by which hypothalamic control of anterior pituitary function is achieved.

The titres of LH, FSH and testosterone were measured simultaneously in blood samples taken at different stages of the seasonal sexual cycle of one adult Soay ram (see figure 7.11). During the first sampling period the testes fully regressed; blood levels of LH, FSH and testosterone were very low. As the testes began to develop, blood samples revealed high FSH titres, probably associated with the restoration of spermatogenesis (see § 7.2); these followed a "pulsatile" pattern. One single large pulse of LH, which was followed by a transient rise in testosterone was also apparent. During the mating season when the testes were full size, blood FSH levels had declined, but many LH "pulses" were present, each one being associated with a sharp rise in blood testosterone titre.

The pulses of gonadotropin release are not unique to this situation. Rapid blood sampling has revealed that several other anterior pituitary hormones show similar fluctuations in titre. The best explanation for these findings is that the hormones concerned are being released in "packets" from the pituitary, thus producing "peak" blood titres; the characteristic exponential decay curves after each peak, coincide with the known half-lives of the hormone in blood.

But why does the pituitary release its hormones in this episodic manner? It is reasonable to suspect that pulsatile secretion of hypothalamic releasing hormones is the probable cause—but their measurement is technically very difficult: they are present in peripheral blood at vanishingly small concentrations, and can only be measured by very sensitive radioimmunoassay in hypophysial portal blood after major (and irreversible) surgery. Experiments on Soay rams, however, have recently provided indirect support for the theory of pulsatile release of Gn-RH (see figure 7.12). Repeated administration of small quantities of Gn-RH at a time of low endogenous levels, produced changes in blood titres of FSH, LH and testosterone similar to those seen during the onset of the mating season. These studies showed also that a single releasing hormone, Gn-RH, can produce different effects on pituitary release of FSH and LH, but the mechanism is unknown.

If hypothalamic releasing hormones are released in pulses, it will provide yet another example of the "neural" characteristics of neurosecretion. Indeed, it is possible that control of anterior pituitary function is dependent on the *frequency* rather than the *amplitude* of such discharges of releasing hormone—in a way directly analogous to nervous modulation.

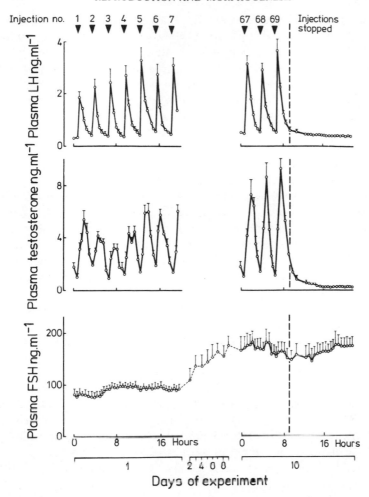

Figure 7.12 The effect of seven injections of 100 ng Gn-RH each day for 9 days and on the tenth day (indicated by arrows) during the inactive stage of the breeding season in a Soay ram. After Lincoln, G. A. (1979) *J. Endocr.*, **80**, 133–140.

7.5 Pregnancy

Viviparity is a reproductive strategy that has evolved independently in numerous diverse animal groups. Among the vertebrates, every class except birds and jawless fish (Agnatha) contains at least one viviparous species. It is in the eutherian mammals, however, that viviparity has been universally adopted and most highly developed.

The retention of young within the body of the mother obviously has required the adoption of a variety of physiological mechanisms not found in the non-pregnant state. How does the maternal organism know when to initiate, and when to terminate these changes in its physiology? The necessary "information" takes the form of hormonal messages allowing coordination of the relationship between fetus and mother. Some selected aspects of the endocrinology of pregnancy are discussed below.

7.5.1   Establishment of pregnancy

It has been suggested that with the evolution of pregnancy in mammals, progesterone was first elevated to the status of a true hormone, rather than a mere intermediate of steroid biosynthesis (see figures 2.9; 2.10). Certainly it is true in all mammals that progesterone, secreted by the maternal corpus luteum, is essential for the early stages of pregnancy. The means by which adequate secretion of progesterone is assured varies considerably in different species. In some (e.g. most marsupials) the gestation period is no longer than an infertile oestrous cycle; no mechanism is required therefore to prolong the life-span of the corpus luteum. In most eutherian mammals, however, some "rescue" of the corpus luteum is necessary. The luteal phase of the oestrous cycle has to be greatly extended, and the return of ovarian cyclicity and ovulation delayed throughout a relatively long gestation period.

In those species where corpus luteum regression is caused by a uterine luteolysin (§ 7.4.1), the presence of a young embryo within the uterus somehow neutralises the lytic effect: either $PGF_2\alpha$ release is prevented, or luteal tissue is made more resistant to it. Often the signal from the embryo which allows maternal recognition of pregnancy seems to be generated prior to any attachment of the blastocyst. The nature of the signal in most cases is still unknown, but recent work with sows suggests that oestrogens produced by blastocysts (as early as day 12 of gestation, or 6 days before implantation in this species) exert both "antiluteolytic" and luteotropic (supportive) influences on the maternal corpus luteum.

In primates, the developing embryo begins secreting a luteotropic hormone—chorionic gonadotropin—at about the time of implantation. Human blastocysts implant about 6 days after conception, and thus generate luteotropic stimuli before corpus luteum regression would be expected in an infertile cycle.

It is apparent then that some of the very earliest actions of the fetus are to usurp control of its mother's ovaries by endocrine means, to secure a progestational environment. This step toward independence—or *fetal autonomy*—is taken further during later pregnancy. In early pregnancy, maternal oophorectomy (ovary removal) results in abortion, due to progesterone withdrawal; it can be prevented by exogenous progesterone administration. In several species, however, the dependence on maternal production of progesterone diminishes as pregnancy progresses, because the fetus establishes an independent supply by placental progesterone biosynthesis.

7.5.2 Progesterone-binding proteins

As we have seen, there is a requirement for a high progesterone titre during pregnancy. In pregnant women and guinea pigs, the level of this hormone is 100-fold greater than in the non-pregnant state. It might be imagined that this would be achieved by increasing the rate of progesterone synthesis. Indeed, this does occur in many species (including the human), partly by forming more corpora lutea—the corpora lutea of pregnancy— and partly because of placental progesterone production. Pregnant guinea pigs (and some other hystricomorph rodents, e.g. coypu) have evolved an alternative strategy in which the rate of degradation of progesterone is greatly decreased during pregnancy. This is associated directly with an increased concentration in the plasma of a special progesterone binding protein: its function is to bind progesterone tightly and thus reduce the rate of its removal from the circulation (see also § 3.4.1).

7.5.3 Parturition

The last 15 years has witnessed a large increase in published information concerning the mechanism of parturition. Large gaps in our understanding of this process still remain, however, and predictably, the picture that emerges is blurred by the apparently numerous species differences.

For parturition to occur, the uterus must undergo two spectacular changes in function: the myometrial muscle, relatively quiescent and supportive during pregnancy, must become vigorously contractile; the uterine cervix, firm and unyielding, which has successfully retained the conceptus until term, must within a few hours become soft and compliant. Both changes are obligatory: active uterine contractions are futile in the absence of cervical "ripening" and if sufficiently provoked (pharmacologically) will lead to uterine rupture rather than a forced cervical dilatation.

It might reasonably be supposed that these drastic reversals in uterine behaviour would be controlled by the mother, but recent research has shown that supposition to be false; the process of parturition is in large measure initiated by the fetus.

Several apparently unrelated pieces of evidence had been available for some time that were compatible with this view. In horses the gestation period is 340 days, but if a mule fetus is carried, gestation is 355 days; in humans, the presence of an anencephalic fetus (severe maldeveloped brain and CNS) is often associated with prolonged pregnancy. Ewes which feed on the skunk cabbage, *Veratrum californicum*, during early pregnancy are affected by an alkaloid in the plant that produces several fetal deformities, particularly in the hypothalamus and pituitary, and gestation is greatly prolonged.

Observations on these "experiments of Nature" led Professor G. C. Liggins to seek direct evidence of fetal involvement in sheep parturition. His group established that ablation of the fetal pituitary *in utero* resulted in prolonged gestation; this outcome was preventable if ACTH or cortisol were infused into the fetal circulation. These experiments, and many others involving several species, strongly indicate that the onset of parturition is a response to a signal originating in the fetus, related to some unidentified maturational event in the fetal hypothalamo-pituitary-adrenocortical axis.

The role of fetal cortisol in the final days of gestation is best understood in the sheep (see figures 7.13 and 7.14). Enzymes capable of converting

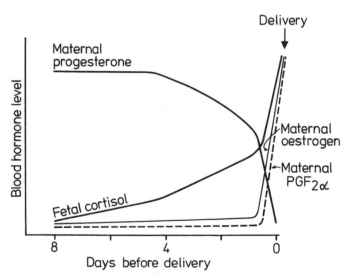

Figure 7.13 Changes in the titres of cortisol in fetal blood and of progesterone, oestrogen and $PGF_2\alpha$ in maternal blood, in relation to the time of parturition of sheep. From Challis, J. R. G., in *Reproduction in Mammals*, Vol. 7 (C. R. Austin and R. V. Short, eds.) C.U.P., 109, Cambridge, 1979.

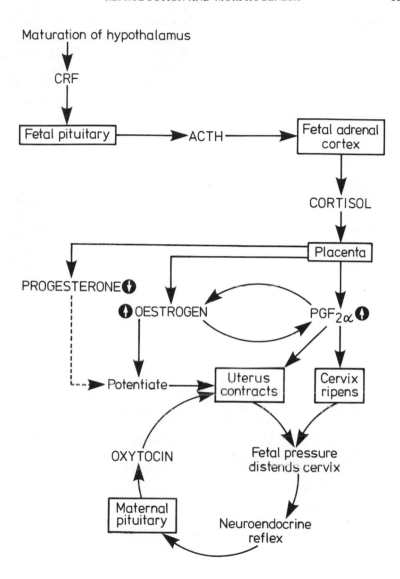

Figure 7.14 Scheme showing the cascade of interrelated events occurring during parturition (based on data mainly from studies on sheep). The signal for onset of parturition is generated by the fetus. $PGF_2\alpha$ has a crucial role, in stimulating uterine contraction and cervical dilatation.

progesterone to oestrogen are induced in placental tissues by cortisol; consequently placental production of progesterone diminishes, and oestrogen levels rise. Progesterone is known in many species to reduce myometrial contractility, probably by hyperpolarizing the smooth muscle membrane potential, and falling titres of progesterone remove this "block". Conversely, oestrogens stimulate myometrial contraction. Rising fetal cortisol output also stimulates placental synthesis and release of a prostaglandin, $PGF_2\alpha$, which plays a central role in parturition. $PGF_2\alpha$ increases oestrogen biosynthesis, by inducing the "aromatization" enzymes (see figure 2.9, and § 7.3). Oestrogens in turn stimulate $PGF_2\alpha$ release. This is, then, another positive feedback loop. $PGF_2\alpha$ probably also contributes to the decline in progesterone, especially in those species like the rabbit and the goat in which an active corpus luteum is essential throughout pregnancy, and the mechanism involved may be similar to that of "non-pregnant" luteolysis (see figure 7.10). Significantly, however, $PGF_2\alpha$ is a potent stimulator of uterine smooth muscle, and—equally important—induces cervical ripening. Uterine contraction, and cervical distension provoke the release of maternal oxytocin, by the neuro-endocrine reflex already discussed (§ 7.1). Oxytocin in turn stimulates further uterine contraction. This positive feedback loop is finally broken as the fetus leaves the birth canal.

This chain of events (see figure 7.14) initiated by the fetal endocrine machinery, while intricate enough, is only part of the story. The perinatal rise in fetal cortisol induces the formation of a fetal lung surfactant, ensuring successful alveolar inflation and air-breathing after birth. The fall in progesterone titre at parturition removes the block exerted on maternal α-lactalbumin synthesis, which is a key reaction in lactogenesis. The fetus thus secures its future food source. Nor is the endocrine communication between fetus and mother entirely severed by parturition. Maternal prolactin output, which controls the level of milk secretion, is quantitatively related to the number of suckling stimuli generated by the newborn. This neuroendocrine reflex is additional to that for milk-ejection (§ 7.1); the suckling infant thus controls both the size and time of delivery of its milk supply.

7.6 Invertebrates

Invertebrates show a wide range of body form and habit and their evolutionary relationships are often obscure. Their endocrine systems vary greatly in structure, even within phyla, and show major differences in function. Nevertheless, the processes of reproduction (from sexual differentiation to gamete emission) are essentially similar in all animals, and hormones control many of these processes. We shall discuss some of the stages of reproductive development and associated endocrine strategies with reference to different invertebrate groups. It should be stressed however, that this treatment will not be comprehensive, nor should it be assumed that the hormonal mechanisms of animals chosen to exemplify particular points are necessarily representative of those in *all* invertebrates; the variations in endocrine control and their degree of involvement in invertebrate functions are too great to allow such generalizations.

7.6.1 *The integrative role of the neurosecretory system*

Reproductive effort must be initiated only when environmental conditions are such that chances of success are high; at a suitable stage of development of the individual, and at the right time of year. The relationship between neurosecretory cells and the central nervous system has already been discussed, and it is not surprising, therefore, that the neuroendocrine system often plays a central role in coordinating environmental information and reproductive activity. Invertebrate neurosecretory cells are often scattered within the nervous system and different populations of cells may fulfil different integrative functions; their combined actions may be analogous with those of the vertebrate hypothalamus (§ 7.1). Collectively, they respond to exteroceptive and interoceptive stimuli, including feedback information from hormones. Our knowledge of feedback mechanisms in invertebrates is, however, fragmentary.

7.6.2 *Sexual differentiation in crustaceans*

In many invertebrates, the primordial gonad of genetic females autodifferentiates into an ovary, but in males, a masculinizing factor is required for testis development. The masculinizing factor is often hormonal and its late intervention or withdrawal may explain sex reversal in hermaphrodites but it is likely that both masculinizing and feminizing factors are produced in some invertebrates. In crustaceans, an androgenic gland (figure 6.3) controls sexual differentiation by exerting a masculinizing influence on the sex organs and those tissues showing secondary sexual characters.

In immature (undifferentiated) crustacea, the sexes cannot be distinguished, but when sexual differentiation begins secondary sexual characters start to appear and in many species their full development is not complete until after gonadal maturity. The undifferentiated stages of both sexes contain primordial vasa deferentia to which are attached rudimentary androgenic glands. These fail to develop in genetic females but in males they enlarge to form solid strands of cells lying between the muscles which move the last pair of walking legs. The cells of the glands secrete in a holocrine fashion, emptying their entire contents into the blood.

Surgical removal of the androgenic glands from young males causes oocytes, rather than spermatocytes, to develop from primary germ cells— but removal of the entire gland is difficult and usually the remnants regenerate and switch development back from oocytes to sperms. If androgenic glands from young males are implanted into females, the ovaries regress rapidly and transform into functional testes. Such masculinized females also behave as males and will copulate with normal females. The androgenic gland controls the development of secondary sexual characters in the male, but female characteristics are not induced merely by the absence of androgenic gland hormone; ovarian hormones exert a positive influence on their development. The chemical nature of the androgenic hormone is uncertain, although it has been suggested that it may be a steroid; testosterone propionate will mimic its action on the ovaries, and the androgenic gland of lobsters is capable of producing testosterone from androstenedione. It is thus possible that the androgenic gland produces a sex steroid but other work has suggested that the hormone may be a protein.

It is likely that intersexes and hermaphroditism in crustacea involve changes in androgenic gland activity. In protandric hermaphrodites, sex reversal is caused by regeneration of the androgenic gland under the influence of gonad-inhibiting hormone from the eye-stalk X-organ-sinus gland complex (figure 6.3). Similarly, the parasite, *Sacculina*, induces feminization in male crabs by causing atrophy of the androgenic glands. This is often referred to as "parasitic castration" but, in fact, there is no castration; the testes may atrophy slightly and often contain oocytes. As the titre of androgenic hormone declines, progressive metamorphosis of the testes into ovaries induces increasingly feminine characters at each moult.

Interestingly, insects have direct genetic control over sex differentiation—except the glow-worm, *Lampyris*, where paired endocrine glands associated with the testes appear to exert a masculinizing action similar to that of the crustacean androgenic gland.

7.6.3   *Growth versus reproduction*
It is self-evident that reproduction should not be attempted until an animal is sufficiently grown to ensure success: we recognize sexually

immature stages in all animals. Towards this end, in many invertebrates hormonal mechanisms ensure a temporal separation of somatic and reproductive growth. In gastropod molluscs and arthropods a balanced synergism between hormones controls somatic and reproductive growth, but in non-nereid polychaetes (see below) and *Octopus*, gonadotropic hormones are only produced at the end of somatic growth. In *Hydra*, the nemertine *Lineus*, and nereid polychaetes, however, somatic growth is stimulated by neurosecretions whose other actions include inhibition of gametogenesis; reproduction proceeds only at the end of somatic growth when these neurosecretions are withdrawn.

Polychaetes Regeneration of amputated caudal segments and reproduction in the polychaete worm, *Nereis*, have been studied extensively. The brain produces a single hormone which promotes regenerative segment proliferation (= somatic growth) and at high concentrations inhibits sexual maturation. The hormone is thought to be produced in cerebral neurosecretory cells some of whose axon tracts terminate close to the neural lamella on the floor of the brain while others run to the infracerebral gland which is closely applied to this region of the brain; additionally it contains intrinsic neurosecretory and glandular epithelial cells. This organization suggests that the infracerebral gland is, in part, a neurohaemal organ for brain neurosecretions. However, when brain hormones are referred to in annelids, their precise source is uncertain.

Experiments involving brain removal and reimplantation in *Nereis* (figure 3.2) suggest that sexual maturation is regulated by a progressive decrease in brain hormone release; as hormone levels decline, segment proliferation (somatic growth) slows and eventually stops, while gametogenesis begins (see figure 7.15). In *Nereis*, sexual development involves a metamorphic change to a more active swimming form—the heteronereis. *Nereis* is monotelic (it breeds only once in its lifetime) and the death of the heteronereis follows soon after spawning when it has fulfilled its function of gamete dispersal. The withdrawal of brain hormone thus commits the worm to a "suicidal" path.

A chemical isolated from maturing nereid oocytes is able to inhibit the release of brain hormone. The active material is of low molecular weight and appears to contain amino acids but is not destroyed by proteolytic enzymes; its chemical identity is thus unknown. It is proposed that this substance forms part of a feedback mechanism whereby developing oocytes *inhibit* the activity of the brain (a *negative* feedback loop) but

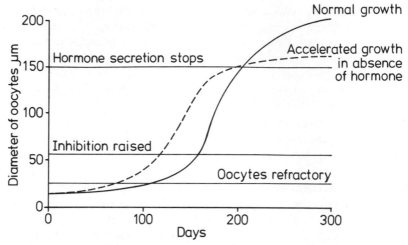

Figure 7.15 The control of oocyte growth in nereid polychaetes. Normal oocyte growth occurs in response to the gradual withdrawal of brain hormone. Removal of the brain causes accelerated but abnormal oocyte growth, suggesting that low titres of brain hormone are essential for normal oocyte growth and vitellogenesis. After Clark; from Highnam, K. C. and Hill, L., in *The Comparative Endocrinology of the Invertebrates*, Edward Arnold, 68, 1977.

consequently *accelerate* further oocyte development (a *positive* feedback loop). The initiation of brain hormone withdrawal, which allows gametogenesis to begin, is probably controlled by photoperiod and temperature.

In non-nereid polychaetes, removal of the brain *inhibits* gametogenesis; the brain exerts a gonadotropic influence. These polychaetes are polytelic and this may suggest an explanation for these endocrine differences. In *Nereis*, regeneration is prevented during sexual maturation because the brain hormone is present at too low a concentration: this is appropriate since regenerated segments could not contribute to future fecundity. In polytelic polychaetes, regeneration is not prevented during oocyte development, presumably because regenerated segments will contribute to future fecundity. Thus, although nereids are unusual amongst polychaetes in suppressing segment regeneration during reproductive development they show, with the polytelic forms, how hormones can regulate the switch from somatic to reproductive growth.

7.6.4 *Vitellogenesis and oocyte maturation*

Incorporation of yolk into developing oocytes is usually associated with their increase in size. This can be measured easily and has therefore been studied intensively. Not surprisingly, endocrine control of the synthesis of yolk precursors (vitellogenesis) and yolk deposition is common in invertebrates; the competition for energy between somatic and reproductive development is most intense at this stage.

Vitellogenesis and yolk deposition in insects In insects which live for only a short time as adults (Lepidoptera commonly) the female emerges with

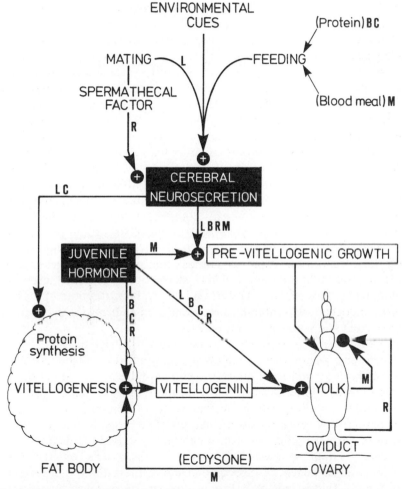

Figure 7.16 Schematic illustration of the endocrine control of reproduction in five insects; Locusts, L; Blowflies, B; *Rhodnius*, R; Mosquitoes, M; and Colorado beetle, C.

almost fully developed oocytes and the *adult* endocrine system does not control egg development. This is appropriate because in these insects the female's main concern is to mate and deposit eggs. The timing of reproductive effort is thus fixed, in the sense that it must occur as soon as possible; many of these adults do not eat. In other insects, vitellogenesis is controlled by juvenile hormone(s) from the corpora allata, often with cerebral neurosecretions acting synergistically (figure 7.16).

In the mosquito, however, it is thought that ingestion of a blood meal releases a brain hormone which stimulates α-ecdysone production by the ovaries; the fat body converts this steroid to β-ecdysone (figure 2.11) and vitellogenesis is stimulated. There is controversy concerning this possible vitellogenic role of ecdysone in mosquitoes; large amounts of injected steroid—many times the physiological levels—are needed to *sustain* vitellogenesis and ecdysone cannot *initiate* vitellogenesis in fat bodies from unfed (non-vitellogenic) females. Nevertheless, ecdysteroids are found in the ovaries of many insects, and ecdysone is usually the major component. It is thought however, that they are concerned with oocyte development and subsequent embryonic processes rather than events outside the ovary. Indeed, it is only in the mosquito that ovarian ecdysone enters the blood. For example, in the locust, the peak of ovarian ecdysone synthesis occurs just before ovulation—when vitellogenesis in the fat body, and yolk deposition in the oocytes, are already complete. In this insect, the follicle cells which surround each oocyte synthesize the ecdysone and provide the newly laid eggs with a large pool of maternal ecdysteroid which appears to control the deposition of the serosal and first embryonic cuticles. Subsequently, the embryo develops its own steroidogenic potential when the prothoracic glands (figure 6.1) differentiate at about the time of blastokinesis; endogenously synthesized ecdysone then controls the production of the second and third embryonic cuticles.

The existence of ovarian steroids in insects is intriguing since in the mosquito and locusts their production is dependent on a gonadotropin from the brain; it will be of interest to compare the source and chemical nature of these adult ecdysiotropins with those in larval insects (§ 6.1.1). Ecdysteroids are also produced in the ovaries of a number of crustacea, and comparisons between ovarian steroids of arthropods and vertebrate oestrogens are tempting; in fish, amphibia, and birds, gonadotropins stimulate ovarian synthesis of oestrogen which acts on the liver to stimulate vitellogenesis. Speculation along these lines is premature until the full significance of arthropod ovarian steroids has been established.

With the possible exception of the mosquitoes, vitellogenesis is controlled by juvenile hormone (JH) but, even in mosquitoes, JH is needed to prime the fat body before it can synthesize yolk proteins. In the majority of female insects, JH induces a spectacular increase in the rate of vitellogenesis. In the cockroach *Leucophaea*, this is prevented by pretreatment of the insect with actinomycin D, suggesting that JH controls transcription of a specific mRNA.

Juvenile hormone acts also as a gonadotropin by stimulating yolk deposition in developing oocytes (figure 7.16). In *Rhodnius*, for example, JH induces the formation of spaces between the follicle cells; a condition which is termed *patency*. Patency allows vitellogenins access to the oocyte surface where uptake occurs by pinocytosis. Patency can be demonstrated in oocytes *in vitro* if JH is present in the culture medium; 10^{-7} molar produces a maximum response but an effect is apparent at 10^{-17} molar. The mechanism by which the follicles change shape during patency is not fully understood but colchicine and cytochalasin B, which disrupt cytoskeletal organization, prevent the response to JH. Ouabain also inhibits patency which suggests that a Na^+/K^+-dependent ATP-ase may also be involved. Interestingly, the oocytes from females in which the corpora allata were removed early in adult life do not show a patency response to JH. It appears that the follicle cells must have reached a particular developmental stage and have been primed at an earlier stage by JH before they will respond.

There is some speculation concerning the possible roles of the three known juvenile hormones (figure 2.12). From studies on the differential sensitivity of reproductive and metamorphic processes to influence by the different homologues, it has been proposed that JH III is principally gonadotropic, whereas JH I and II are more potent morphogenetic agents during larval life (§ 7.7.2).

Cyclic development of oocytes in insects   In many insects, the terminal oocyte in each ovariole develops in synchrony with its neighbours and batches of eggs are laid; a new cycle of synchronous oocyte development begins soon after ovulation. Consequently, egg batches are laid at more or less regular intervals.

There is considerable histological evidence which suggests that these reproductive cycles are caused by varying secretory activity of the cerebral neurosecretory cells and/or the corpora allata. In recent studies the corpora allata from female locusts and cockroaches, at different times of the reproductive cycle, have been cultured for short periods so that JH release into the medium could be measured; the corpora allata show cycles of synthetic activity with the same periodicity as the synchronous ovulation of the terminal oocytes.

What is the cause of these cyclic changes in endocrine activity? A large number of environmental factors influence secretory activity; feeding and mating are major stimuli and could initiate the first ovarian cycle. But what causes a decrease in endocrine activity at the end of this and subsequent cycles? The answer to this question is largely unknown but, by analogy with ovarian cycles in vertebrates (§ 7.4.1), it may be that the presence of the developing oocytes causes the insect ovary to produce a hormone which prevents further gonadotropin release. There is some evidence for feedback mechanisms by gonadal hormones in insects but they act in different ways in different insect species; they can inhibit the activity of the cerebral neurosecretory cells and/or the corpora allata, or they can exert localized antigonadotropic effects on immature oocytes (figure 7.16). Stretch receptors in the abdomen may relay information about oocyte development to the brain; in the viviparous cockroach, *Leucophaea*, the developing young in the "uterus" stimulate sensory receptors which act via the brain to inhibit the corpora allata so that the next ovarian cycle is delayed until "parturition". Furthermore, in *Rhodnius* an antigonadotropin is released from groups of neurosecretory cells embedded in the connective tissue sheath around the ovary; these cells may monitor growth of the terminal oocytes by the stretch in the connective tissue sheath. Secretions of these cells are thought to act locally to inhibit development in pre-vitellogenic oocytes. Extracts of the cells prevent the patency response to JH.

Perhaps the terminating process of one cycle triggers off the beginning of the next (cf. § 7.4.1). Certainly, in locusts, oviposition stimulates cerebral neurosecretory activity; the next ovarian cycle begins immediately if food availability and other environmental conditions are favourable.

7.6.5 *Spawning and ovulation*

Many aquatic invertebrates shed their gametes into the external medium for fertilization. It is therefore important that spawning is controlled so that eggs and sperm may come together; temperature and photoperiod may determine the suitable timing. In those invertebrates in which fertilization is internal, ovulation and egg laying must still be coordinated with environmental conditions; hormones play an essential role in these mechanisms. We will discuss two examples; spawning in *Asterias* and the aquatic gastropod molluscs, *Lymnaea* and *Aplysia*.

Starfish The radial nerve in *Asterias* releases a low molecular weight (about 2100) polypeptide neurohormone—shedding hormone—which causes simultaneous spawning of the paired gonads of each arm. In females, injected hormone causes spawning after about 45 minutes. Isolated ovaries respond to such extracts by the dissolution of cementing substances between follicles themselves and between the follicle cells and the oocyte surface, freeing the oocytes and allowing them to be expelled by the contraction of smooth muscle in the ovarian wall. Simultaneously, the oocytes mature by completing their meiotic division. The movement of the follicle cells away from the surface of the oocytes to free them for ovulation is caused by changes in shape of the follicle cells but its mechanism is unknown. Shedding hormone does not stimulate oocyte maturation and ovulation directly; its primary action is to stimulate follicle cell synthesis of a maturation-inducing substance which has been identified as 1-methyladenine. It is this factor from the follicle cells which frees the oocytes and restarts meiosis. The two effects of 1-methyladenine occur at different threshold concentrations; 10^{-7} molar will provoke the resumption of meiosis, whereas 10^{-6} molar is needed to free the oocytes. The mechanisms by which the maturation inducing factor exerts its actions are uncertain.

The radial nerve also produces a hormone which inhibits spawning. Thus spawning may be controlled seasonally by variations in the production of this inhibitory hormone so that gamete shedding is prevented during most of the year by high concentrations of this second hormone. The rationale for such an apparently complicated mechanism is not clear but when female starfish of the same species are kept together in an aquarium, they often show synchronous spawning. It is suggested that the shedding hormone may escape into the sea water and exert a pheromone-like effect on other females (this is not thought to be the normal route for transfer of the hormone to the ovary). Since the species specificity of shedding hormone is poor (or absent in most cases), the inhibiting factor may prevent interspecific interactions; two species of starfish may be kept together and yet spawn at different times. In nature, the inhibitory hormone from the radial nerve may thus serve to prevent inappropriate spawning.

Gastropod molluscs Two species of aquatic gastropod molluscs have been much studied—*Lymnaea*, a freshwater pulmonate, and the marine opisthobranch, *Aplysia*. Both possess ovulation hormones which are the products of neurosecretory cells in the nervous system. In *Lymnaea*, the

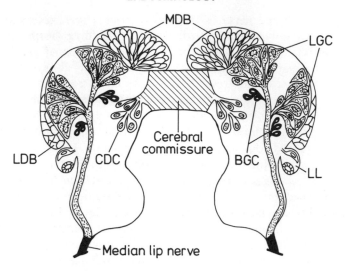

Figure 7.17 Diagrammatic section through the cerebral ganglia of the fresh water pulmonate snail *Lymnaea*. LGC and BGC = light and bright green neurosecretory cells; CDC = caudo dorsal cells; LL = lateral lobes; MDB and LDB = medial and lateral dorsal bodies. The sites of release for the LGC and BGC are the periphery of the median lip nerves, and that for the CDC is the cerebral commissure. After Geraerts, W. P. M. and Joosse, J. (1975) *Gen. Comp. Endocr.*, **27**, 450–464.

lateral lobes of the cerebral ganglia are thought to act as integration centres for the control of reproduction. They stimulate vitellogenesis and egg laying indirectly by acting through the dorsal bodies and caudodorsal cells (CDC), and inhibit somatic growth via the LGC (figure 7.17). The CDC produce an ovulation hormone. At low doses, hormone injection releases oocytes from the ovotestis but higher doses are needed for the packaging of oocytes into the characteristic gelatinous egg masses which are extruded 2 h later. The ovulation hormone is a low molecular weight peptide and may act by stimulating muscular contractions of the walls of the acini (lobules) in the ovotestis; a chronic action is also suggested by the rapid degeneration of mature oocytes after surgical removal of the CDC.

The CDC cells appear to respond rapidly and directly to changes in photoperiod and temperature; a sudden rise in temperature (or oxygenation) may induce ovulation within minutes by a neuroendocrine reflex. Photoperiod, however, is the most powerful environmental influence on the activity of the CDC. Long days (16 h light : 8 h dark) accelerate female development and increase egg production 10–20 fold compared with short days (8 h light: 16 h dark). This stimulatory effect is so great that, in the laboratory, starved "long-day" snails continue to lay eggs until their reserves are exhausted, and they die prematurely compared with "short-day" snails which survive starvation for long periods; the reserves of short-day snails are conserved by the cessation of egg production. Thus the response of the CDC to environmental factors enables the snail to exploit its habitat to the full. The ponds inhabited by *Lymnaea* have only sparse areas which are rich in oxygen, have high temperatures, and are thus rich in algae (food for the newly hatched snails); it is important, therefore, that eggs are laid during the summer months in such locations.

In the sea hare, *Aplysia*, an ovulation hormone released from neurosecretory cells—so-called "bag cells"—clustered around the visceral ("abdominal") ganglion causes the ovotestis to release mature oocytes which are later packaged into strings of gelatinous capsules in the reproductive tract. Ovulation occurs within 1 min of hormone injection but egg strings are laid 30–60 min later. The hormone initiates some aspects of egg laying behaviour directly; if the hermaphrodite duct is ligatured close to the ovotestis, so that oocytes cannot be packaged, hormone injection still inhibits some aspects of feeding behaviour, but the characteristic head weaving movements associated with extrusion of the egg strings, does not occur. This suggests that while head weaving behaviour is an indirect effect of the hormone (probably triggered by the movement of the eggs along the reproductive tract), feeding inhibition is a direct effect of the hormone on the central nervous system.

Under normal conditions, ovulation in *Aplysia* is probably initiated during mating, afferent stimuli to the bag cells travelling by the pleurovisceral connectives. When these connective nerves are cut, *Aplysia* shows a much reduced level of spontaneous egg laying activity. Removal of the bag cells (by ablation of the visceral ganglion) does not, however, completely prevent egg laying and an alternative source of ovulation hormone may exist. Indeed, some workers claim that glands associated with the reproductive tract contain a biologically active substance which is chemically similar to bag cell peptide. The full significance of this second peptide is unknown.

The electrophysiology of bag cells and CDC has been studied extensively. In both *Aplysia* and *Lymnaea*, the cells are electrotonically coupled so that they fire synchronously—in *Lymnaea* this synchrony extends to the left and right clusters of CDC in the cerebral ganglia. This ensures coordinated massive release of ovulation hormone, by recruiting all cells in the population(s). Although the cells are usually electrically silent, they can be stimulated electrically to undergo spontaneous bursting activity, often showing a prolonged period of afterdischarge. In *Lymnaea*, the release of ovulation hormone has been demonstrated during this afterdischarge *in vitro*, and, in *Aplysia*, spontaneous bursting activity of the bag cells *in vivo* correlates with egg laying some 30 min later. Interestingly, in *Lymnaea*, the afterdischarge of the CDC is dependent on the previous light regime of the snail; afterdischarge is only observed in CDC from long-day snails.

These exciting studies may lead to a better understanding of the relationship between electrical activity and neurohormone secretion. One attractive hypothesis is that bursting activity, which is common to many neurosecretory cells, causes hormone release by depolarization of the axon terminals, which allows calcium entry and stimulates hormone secretion (§ 2.3.1).

7.7 Metamorphosis

Many animals exist as two or more morphologically (and physiologically) distinct free-living stages during their post-embryonic development—metamorphosis is the transformation from one body form to another. The intervention of metamorphosis in an animal's development allows the exploitation of different habitats and often involves dramatic differences in feeding, locomotion and behaviour. We have already seen how metamorphosis in the polychaete *Nereis* is regulated by a brain hormone, and in higher animals hormones are equally important—only in a few animals, however, is their involvement understood in any depth.

7.7.1 *Vertebrates*

Euryhaline fish (see § 8.2.4) occupy different habitats during their life, and those such as the eels and lampreys show dramatic metamorphic changes—but in others, such as the salmon, these are less marked. These changes are probably controlled by pituitary and thyroid hormones, but it is the endocrinology of amphibian metamorphosis which is best understood; especially that of the anurans, *Rana* and *Xenopus*.

Anurans   The familiar changes which occur during the transformation of anuran tadpoles into adult frogs and toads are dramatic: the fully aquatic larva without lungs or limbs, suddenly grows legs, crawls onto land and becomes terrestrial. Environmental factors such as nutritional state, temperature, degree of crowding, chemical quality of the water and photoperiod may all interact to *initiate* metamorphosis but the dominant endocrine influences are exerted by thyroid hormones and prolactin.

Tadpoles undergo precocious metamorphosis when fed extracts of thyroid glands or when injected with TSH (thyroid stimulating hormone). These experiments suggest that although the immediate cause of metamorphosis may be the changing pattern of thyroid activity, this is regulated by the output of TSH from the pituitary. In premetamorphic tadpoles (figure 7.18) there are low levels of T_4 and T_3 (tetraiodothyronine

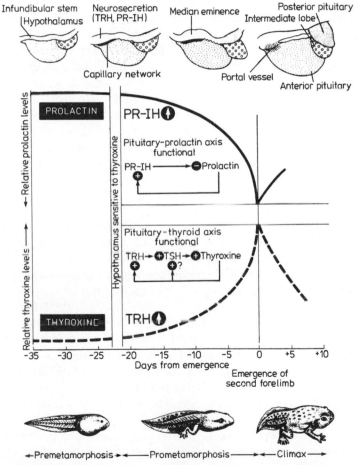

Figure 7.18 The role of hormones in the growth and development of the tadpole of the frog. After Bentley, P. J., in *Comparative Vertebrate Endocrinology*, C.U.P., 372, 1976.

and triiodothyronine; figure 2.13) in the blood. (The origin of T_3 is not clear since it is not synthesized in the thyroid, and deiodinating enzymes from amphibia do not produce T_3 from T_4). There is circumstantial evidence that at this stage thyronines exert an adult-type negative feedback control of TSH secretion. Coincident with these low levels of thyronines, the prolactin content of the blood is high; the prolactin release-inhibiting hormone (PR-IH) is not present. At this stage the larva can be thought of as stabilized; high levels of prolactin and low levels of thyronines stimulate larval growth.

At the onset of the prometamorphic stage (figure 7.18), the differentiation of the hypothalamic neurosecretory system and the pituitary begins, and the control of TSH release changes; thyronines exert a positive feedback influence by stimulating release of TRH (thyroid releasing hormone) from the hypothalamus. This is the signal for the onset of metamorphosis; increasing titres of T_4 and T_3 stimulate further development of the pituitary, and the portal vessels (see figure 7.18). One consequence of this is the release of PR-IH so that as thyronine levels increase, prolactin levels decrease (figure 7.18).

These changing patterns of hormone titre initiate gross morphological changes; specifically larval tissues, like the tail, which have grown and been maintained under the influence of prolactin, are resorbed, and adult tissues, such as the limbs, differentiate (see also § 3.3.1). Prolactin and thyroid hormones control metamorphosis by a balanced synergism; prolactin opposes the actions of thyronines in initiating tail resorption, for example, so that the changes in titre of both hormones are necessary for controlled metamorphic development.

Thyroidal stimulation of metamorphosis must act through the differentiation of the hypothalamo-pituitary axis and not simply by a direct peripheral action on sensitive tissues; in the absence of PR-IH, high titres of prolactin would prevent metamorphosis as, indeed, do injections of prolactin (or larval pituitary grafts) into larvae. The positive feedback of thyronines on the hypothalamus clearly leads to a climax situation (figure 7.18); metamorphosis is completed and further control of TRH release in the adult is by a *negative* feedback, but the mechanism by which this changed responsiveness of the hypothalamus/pituitary occurs is unknown.

Urodeles Metamorphic change in urodeles (newts and salamanders) is less pronounced than in anurans; the lifestyles of the larva and adult are often not so different. The pattern of endocrine control of metamorphosis in urodeles is similar to that of anurans, but there are some important differences. Leg growth is not thyroxine dependent, and the switch to negative feedback of TRH which occurs in postmorphic anurans is not seen in urodeles; thyroid activity persists in adults.

The American spotted newt, *Notophthalamus*, undergoes two metamorphic changes. The first, from aquatic larva to the adult, or red *eft* (see also §8.2.3), and a second when the terrestrial eft returns to water to breed; this second metamorphosis is associated with a reduction in thyroid activity and an increase in prolactin secretion.

A number of urodeles are *neotenic*: they retain larval characters but breed while in the larval form. Some, like the familiar axolotl, *Ambystoma mexicanum*, and the mud puppy, *Necturus*, do not normally show a metamorphosis, although the axolotl (but not *Necturus*) responds to exogenous thyroid hormone by metamorphosing into an adult salamander. Other neotenic species like the tiger salamander, *Ambystoma tigrinum*, show a facultative neoteny since both terrestrial (metamorphosed) and aquatic morphs (neotenes) can be found breeding in the same pond. When these neotenic tiger salamanders are brought into the laboratory, they undergo spontaneous metamorphosis; this is most likely a "stress" effect but long photoperiods and high temperatures which enhance thyroid function also stimulate metamorphosis.

The development of reproductive potential in neotenes is most likely a consequence of high levels of prolactin secretion—the hormone is a gonadotropin in amphibia (as it is in mammals). Ovine prolactin enhances ovulation in females and the development of androgen-dependent sex accessory structures in male tiger salamander newts.

7.7.2 *Insects*

Although the metamorphosis of a tadpole into an adult frog may be regarded as dramatic, the development of a moth or butterfly from what can often be an inconspicuous caterpillar is even more remarkable. In holometabolous insects like these, the intervention of the pupal stage has allowed increasing and divergent evolution of the two morphs to different lifestyles; the caterpillar or grub is an active, crawling, eating and growing stage which gives way to the flying adult which takes on the responsibility for reproduction (see also §7.6.3). Hemimetabolous insects show a less dramatic metamorphosis; although larval moults introduce gradual changes towards the adult, the final moult allows the full development of functional wings and other adult characters.

In holometabolous insects, adult tissues develop largely from the growth in the pupal stage of small islands of tissue (imaginal discs) which are present in the larval body, but quiescent, since embryogenesis. In hemimetabolous species, however, the adult tissues form from the same cells (or their descendants) that produced the larval body. Evidently these cells carry a dual genetic potentiality; to produce larval or adult body patterns. In both groups of insects, metamorphosis is controlled by juvenile hormone (JH) from the corpora allata.

The role of JH during metamorphosis can best be illustrated by considering Sir Vincent Wigglesworth's experiments on the reduviid bug, *Rhodnius*. Wigglesworth noted that a few larvae moulted when they had been decapitated towards the end of the critical period (§6.1.1) and some of these showed varying degrees of precocious development; adult characters such as partial differentiation of the wings and genitalia were expressed. The effect diminished through the critical period and by its end, none of the decapitated insects which moulted showed this precocious development.

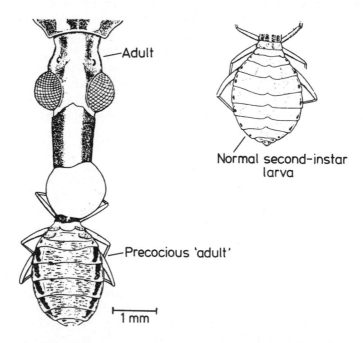

Figure 7.19 A precocious "adult" *Rhodnius* formed from a first-stage larva by joining it parabiotically to the head of a moulting fifth-stage larva. A normal second-stage larva is shown for comparison. After Wigglesworth, V. B. (1940) *J. Exp. Biol.*, **17**, 201–222.

In his classical parabiosis experiments (figure 7.19), Wigglesworth went on to show that larval characters are maintained, and metamorphosis is inhibited, by a humoral factor (JH) from the corpora allata; precocious metamorphosis in the decapitation experiments resulted from the removal of these glands. Thus, Wigglesworth concluded that in hemimetabolous insects, metamorphosis in early instars is prevented by high titres of JH, but during successive instars the JH titre decreases gradually allowing some development towards the adult; in the final stage larva, JH is not secreted and metamorphosis occurs (figure 7.19). Similar effects of JH have been demonstrated in many other species. In holometabolous insects, allatectomy (ablation of the corpora allata) of young larvae induces precocious pupation and, ultimately, small adults.

Recently it has been possible to measure JH by bioassay or RIA (§ 3.2.2). In general, these methods have confirmed the interpretation of earlier experiments; JH titre is high during larval stages and low or absent during the last larval instar (or during pupation). The mechanisms by which these changes in JH titre are controlled are not clear. The control of the activity of the corpora allata is complex; it is innervated by both conventional and neurosecretory neurones and their relative importance in influencing secretory activity varies from species to species, and humoral control cannot be excluded. (The possible role of JH esterases and binding proteins has been discussed in §3.4.3).

In general, the brain exerts a central role in controlling the corpora allata and the cerebral neurosecretory cells may play a prominent part. In some insects these neurosecretory cells are subject to negative feedback control by JH and ecdysone; the latter may, in part, be an explanation for the critical period required to activate the prothoracic glands (§ 6.1.1). Our knowledge of feedback mechanisms in insects is, however, inadequate to generate a general theory of corpus allatum control.

An interesting example of control of JH activity is shown by the tobacco hornworm, *Manduca*. In this insect, the initiation of pupation depends on the weight of the caterpillar; once it has achieved a weight of 5 g (some form of allometry must determine this) the corpora allata become inactive and pupation occurs at the next moult.

The morphogenetic effect of JH is dependent on its time of release or experimental application; for it to be fully effective it must be present early in the instar. The target tissues are sensitive to JH for only a limited period which differs from tissue to tissue and between instars; once this is passed, even large doses are unable to influence the developmental outcome of the next moult.

The action of JH should not be envisaged as simply *negative* or inhibitory; it exerts a *positive* influence in that it promotes larval characters. Indeed, JH treatment can cause de-differentiation of epidermal cells when adults are made to moult by injecting ecdysone (or by parabiosis with moulting larvae); they produce a second *adult* cuticle when only ecdysone is injected, but a new larval cuticle when pre-treated with JH. These observations are of great importance in our understanding of how JH and ecdysone synergistically control insect metamorphosis. The epidermis is a common target tissue for these hormones but the times at which they act upon it are different; JH *determines* (early in the instar) its covert developmental fate which will only be expressed overtly at some later time when ecdysone initiates a moult. Ecdysone can be thought of as playing a permissive role. JH determines how far, and in which direction, epidermal cells will progress along their own intrinsic morphogenetic programme, switching on genes controlling larval pattern and suppressing genes for adult characters, at a time determined by ecdysone release.

CHAPTER EIGHT

IONIC AND OSMOTIC REGULATION

IN ALL ANIMALS THE PHYSICOCHEMICAL PROPERTIES AND COMPOSITION of the cellular and body fluids differ quantitatively and qualitatively from those of the external environment. Even though the osmotic concentration of the body fluid of many marine organisms is similar to sea water, the detailed composition differs markedly. Similarly, within the body the intracellular and extracellular fluids are very different. Animals achieve a homeostasis of their body fluids by:

(i)   the possession, in particular organs and tissues, of membranes whose permeability to different ions may be regulated;
(ii)   the action of pumps which can transport ions against concentration gradients.

In many invertebrates and in all vertebrates the integration of these homeostatic processes is controlled largely by hormones whose target tissues are the integument, the gut and the excretory tubules.

8.1   Invertebrates

There is little information concerning the endocrine control of ionic and osmotic regulation in most non-arthropod invertebrates. One exception is the molluscs where there is histological evidence for the involvement of neurosecretory cells (in various ganglia) in osmotic and ionic regulation, but their role has not been fully established. It is only in crustaceans and insects that clear evidence of hormonal control is available.

8.1.1   Crustacea

In many crustacea, water balance is regulated precisely during the moult cycle. The moment of ecdysis is determined by the uptake of water which increases the size of the animal and splits off the old cuticle. The common shore crab, *Carcinus*, increases its volume by 80 % during a moult, but if its eyestalks are removed the increase is 180 %. This abnormal water uptake is prevented by injecting extracts of the sinus glands and these extracts also reduce the normal uptake of water in intact crabs. This neurosecretory water balance hormone is distinct from the moult inhibiting hormone (§6.1.1) from the sinus gland and the two hormones are released independently. The time of ecdysis is controlled precisely and crabs and lobsters, for example, moult at a time and in a sheltered place of their own choosing; the onset of ecdysis is caused by the lack of release of the water balance hormone and this affords a most important protective mechanism. Removal of the eyestalks from crabs accelerates the onset of ecdysis by increasing water uptake; such crabs exhibit several rapid moults but soon die due to excessive uptake of water. In freshwater decapods there is evidence for the existence of a neurosecretory hormone which regulates ionic flux, especially that of Na^+, independently of the water balance hormones.

8.1.2   *Insects*

Terrestrial insects are extremely well adapted to conserving water, but excess water intake occurs intermittently and has necessitated the development of endocrine mechanisms to deal with this special problem. In most terrestrial insects a diuretic hormone acts on the Malpighian tubules, but the detailed mechanisms and sites of production and release of hormones differ between species.

In locusts, the rate of production of primary urine by the Malpighian tubules is normally more or less equal to the rate of fluid absorption by the rectum. The rates are of the order of $20 \, \mu l \, h^{-1}$. In times of water shortage a minimal amount of fluid is secreted by the tubules, and this is reabsorbed from the rectum. To promote water loss a diuretic hormone produced by the neurosecretory cells in the pars intercerebralis of the brain is released from the neurohaemal storage lobes of the corpora cardiaca. The diuretic hormone increases markedly the rate of urine secretion by the Malpighian tubules and the volume of urine entering the rectum exceeds its absorptive capacity. The effect of the hormone is thus to ensure that excess water is lost in the faeces. The source of this water is the plant material in the diet and it can be considerable—up to $2000 \, \mu l$ each day. It is the act of feeding that elicits the release of the hormone and so in the locust, the endocrine regulation of water balance is a well coordinated system.

In the blood-sucking bug *Rhodnius*, two neurosecretory hormones are released in response to each large meal. Axon terminals close to the abdominal wall release a plasticization hormone which promotes an increase in the water content of the cuticle allowing it to stretch and accommodate the meal. The second hormone is a diuretic hormone produced by 12 neurosecretory cells in the mesothoracic ganglion. The axons of these cells do not form a discrete neurohaemal organ—hormone is released from the surface of the abdominal nerves. Small meals do not cause hormone release; for this to occur, the abdomen must be distended fully. Feeding on warm saline also induces rapid diuresis, so it is clearly abdominal distention itself rather than the quality of the stimuli from the mouthparts which elicits hormone release. Severance of the nerve cord prevents hormone release by preventing information from the stretch receptors in the abdominal wall passing into the neuropile of the thoracic ganglion. The neuropile also receives dendritic branches from the neurosecretory cells and an integrative link must exist within the neuropile so that the neurosecretory cells respond rapidly to abdominal distension. Hormone release is rapid and the Malpighian tubules show maximum diuresis within 2 min of the onset of feeding. This is an example of a neuroendocrine reflex (see §7.1). The stretch receptors in the abdomen adapt only slowly to ensure that the diuretic hormone is released for as long as the blood meal is present in the gut. The half-life of the diuretic hormone in the haemolymph is short so that any hormone circulating in the haemolymph is quickly removed, ensuring that diuresis stops when hormone is no longer released.

The physiology of urine formation in insects has been studied extensively using preparations of Malpighian tubules *in vitro* where the rate of urine production and influence of hormones can be monitored (figure 8.1). Analysis of the composition of the urine is facilitated because urine can be collected free from gut contents. In most insects the flow of urine across the Malpighian tubule cell into the lumen is driven by an electrogenic pump which actively secretes K^+. Primary urine is therefore iso-osmotic to the haemolymph. In some insects, such as *Rhodnius* and the tsetse fly, Na^+ movement may also be involved in urine formation.

There is uncertainty concerning the mode of action of insect diuretic hormone but its stimulatory effect is impressive: in *Rhodnius*, the tubules increase their rate of fluid secretion 600 fold. The hormones in locusts, tsetse fly and *Rhodnius* appear to be small peptides whose action, in common with many other peptide hormones, involves adenylate cyclase. Cyclic AMP mimics the action of diuretic hormones and in *Rhodnius* cAMP levels in the tubules are elevated for 2–4 min after stimulation with

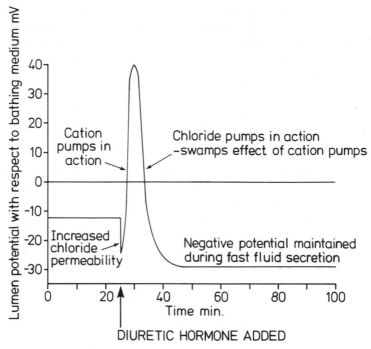

Figure 8.1 Possible explanation for the effects of diuretic hormone upon the transepithelial potential across the Malpighian tubule of *Rhodnius*. After Maddrell, S. H. P. (1971) *Adv. Insect Physiol.*, **8**, 199–331.

diuretic hormone. However, such observations tell us little of the nature of the solute pumps and the protein kinases which activate them. More information has come from measurements of trans-epithelial potential during stimulation with diuretic hormone (figure 8.1). The potentials across resting and stimulated tubules are similar but the net flux of ions in the stimulated state is much greater. The short-lived change in membrane potential caused by diuretic hormone parallels closely the increase in the intracellular levels of cAMP.

The composition of the urine voided finally from the insect depends upon the reabsorption of ions and organic solutes, which occurs both within the hindgut and tubules. There is little information concerning hormonal control of these processes but in herbivores such as locusts there is sufficient K^+ present in the diet to ensure that the haemolymph does not become deficient in this ion. However, in blood-sucking insects such as

Rhodnius, the diet is low in K$^+$ and to maintain rapid rates of urine flow it is essential that K$^+$ is recycled from the primary urine back into the haemolymph as quickly as is possible. In *Rhodnius* this reabsorption occurs in the region of the Malpighian tubule nearest the gut and is stimulated by diuretic hormone. The mechanism is efficient and the K$^+$ concentration falls from 140 mM in the primary urine to 4 mM as the urine passes into the hindgut. In locusts a potentially antidiuretic factor present in the corpora cardiaca increases the rate of fluid reabsorption in rectal preparations *in vitro*. The locust diuretic hormone acts *in vitro* to reduce water uptake from the rectal lumen. However, it is not clear whether such factors function as hormones on the rectum *in vivo*. Some recent studies in locusts have described the presence of a corpus cardiacum hormone, which is released into the haemolymph, and stimulates the active reabsorption of Cl$^-$ from the hindgut lumen. Whether this action is related to the antidiuretic response or is particularly for the conservation of this anion is not clear. Locusts possess efficient mechanisms for reabsorbing cations from the rectal lumen but there is no evidence that these are under hormonal control.

8.2 Vertebrates

Vertebrates occupy a wide spectrum of osmotic environments, ranging from sea, fresh and brackish waters through to arid deserts. Marked differences exist in the availability of water and salts in these environments and the variability within a particular environment can often be pronounced. In many terrestrial vertebrates, their biological design commits them to high rates of evaporative water loss from the skin and respiratory surfaces and their large size prevents them from inhabiting small, moist, enclosed spaces. Water loss can be very high, especially in hot dry air; such losses are often exacerbated in homeotherms by panting or sweating. Additionally, water loss occurs in the faeces and urine, and increases also during lactation or egg laying.

Many vertebrates are aquatic but the ionic and osmotic problems encountered in fresh water are very different from those in sea water. In fresh water, which is hypo-osmotic to the body fluids of all animals, they face osmotic flooding and loss of salts by diffusion across permeable membranes. With the exception of amphibians and, for example, soft-shelled turtles, the skin of most vertebrates is relatively impermeable to water, although in fish the gills are a potential site for water gain and passive salt loss. Salts are obtained in the diet and sodium chloride is taken up actively across amphibian skin and the gills of fishes. The kidney is an important site for water elimination and, although most salts are reabsorbed from urine, some salt loss may continually occur in the urine.

In sea water, which is markedly hyperosmotic to the body fluids of most vertebrates, water is lost by osmosis and salts are gained passively. The exceptions are the hagfish and the coelocanth, which are iso-osmotic, and the elasmobranchs and one known marine amphibian, which maintain hyperosmolarity by retention of urea and sodium chloride in the blood. Marine teleosts maintain water balance by drinking sea water and absorbing the salt (followed by water) across the gut wall. Excess sodium chloride is excreted by special chloride-secreting cells in the gills, and divalent ions such as magnesium, calcium and sulphate are secreted in the urine. Water loss is minimized by a reduction in urine volume. This has been achieved by a reduction in the number of actively filtering nephrons (see also §8.2.4), or by reduction in size or loss of the glomerulus altogether. Some marine fishes are thus said to be aglomerular and in these urine is formed wholly by secretion. If urine is formed by filtration, water loss may be minimized by increased reabsorption of water in the renal tubule, although hypertonicity of the urine cannot be achieved.

Many terrestrial vertebrates live close to or in close association with fresh water, and water balance may be maintained by drinking or by the characteristically amphibian method of absorbing it through the skin. Many amphibians and some reptiles can store urine in a bladder where sodium and other solutes and water may be reabsorbed. Birds and most reptiles lack a urinary bladder and urine refluxes back through the cloaca and up into the hindgut where both salts and water may be taken back into the blood. Salts are gained in the diet and any excess can be excreted by the kidneys and, in many birds and reptiles, by the (nasal) salt-secreting glands.

In all vertebrates, hormones influence osmoregulation by affecting the kidneys, skin, bladder, gills, gut and salt glands by varying degrees in different species; the major hormones involved are the neurohypophysial hormones, adrenocorticosteroids, catecholamines, prolactin and angio-tensin. The actions of these hormones in different vertebrates will now be discussed, but it should be appreciated that many aspects of homeostasis may also be under neural control. There is, for example, considerable evidence that the salt glands in birds secrete in response to stimulation by the autonomic cholinergic system and, in mammals, adrenalin released at nerve endings may restrict blood flow and so affect the homeostatic organs. Indeed, the sweat glands respond to adrenalin released locally from nerves; during exercise, however, it is likely that the sweat glands respond to adrenalin in the circulation.

8.2.1 Mammals

The mammalian kidney is unique amongst vertebrates in producing a hypertonic urine. This ability is important in regulating water loss and is dependent on the activity of nephrons which possess a hairpin-like structure called the loop of Henle. Mammalian nephrons can be classified according to their location in the kidney into three broad categories: superficial and intermediate cortical nephrons, and juxtamedullary, and each category shows considerable heterogeneity of function. Mammalian cortical nephrons have a relatively short loop of Henle whereas those with glomeruli in the juxtaglomerular region have longer loops, about one third of which extend into the medullary pyramids. There is a steady increase in osmotic pressure of mammalian kidney tissue from cortex to the innermost part of the medulla. Chloride pumps in the ascending limb of the loop of Henle create this concentration gradient by the operation of a countercurrent concentrating mechanism which depends for its action on the hairpin configuration. The osmotic gradient in the kidney tissue is maintained by the peritubular capillaries which in juxtaglomerular nephrons, form a hairpin loop, the vasa recta, alongside the loop of Henle and act as a countercurrent exchange mechanism. Solutes diffuse passively into descending and out of ascending vessels; water diffuses out of descending and into ascending vessels. Hypertonicity of medullary tissues is thus maintained. The urine in the descending limb of the loop of Henle becomes more concentrated towards the tip of the loop as it comes into osmotic equilibrium with the kidney tissue, and then becomes more dilute as it travels up the ascending limb due to the action of chloride pumps in the relatively impermeable tubule wall. Concentration of the urine occurs in the collecting ducts as the urine equilibrates osmotically with the kidney tissue on its travel towards the pyramids (figure 8.2); reabsorbed water is removed from medullary tissue by the vasa recta. The rate and pattern of blood flow within the glomeruli and vasa recta play an important part in the regulation of both glomerular filtration rate (GFR) and tubular reabsorption; these represent prime targets for hormone action.

Antidiuretic hormone   Mammals possess an antidiuretic hormone (ADH) and in most this is the octapeptide vasopressin (table 1.2); under the influence of ADH the urine leaving the kidney is markedly hyperosmotic to the body fluids. The osmotic water removed from the primary urine

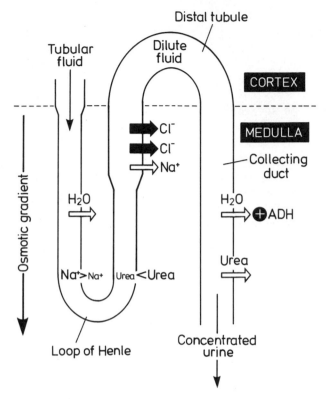

Figure 8.2 Schematic illustration of the operation of the countercurrent concentrating system in the formation of concentrated urine in the mammalian kidney. Active transport of chloride is indicated by the solid arrows, and passive flux by the open arrows. The walls of the ascending limb of the loop of Henle are relatively impermeable to water but the walls of the descending limb and the collecting duct are permeable.

diffuses into the ascending limb of the vasa recta and is transported away from the kidney. The net effect is an increase in volume and osmolarity of the blood. ADH release is influenced by changes in the blood volume and osmolarity (monitored by the hypothalamus) and forms part of a simple closed loop system (§2.3). Haemorrhaging (i.e. marked fall in blood volume) leads to a massive release of ADH; at these high concentrations the hormone may exert a pressor effect, elevating blood pressure by causing the arterioles to contract. Its prime function, however, is to reduce urinary water loss from the kidney tubules, where it increases the water permeability of the collecting duct cells and allows more to pass by osmosis from the lumen of the collecting ducts into the hyperosmotic interstitial fluid surrounding the ducts.

Aldosterone   The Na^+/K^+ balance in mammals is regulated largely by two important adrenocorticosteroids, aldosterone and corticosterone. They reduce sodium excretion and enhance potassium secretion in the saliva and sweat, and aldosterone may also increase Na^+ uptake from the gut—but their most important osmoregulatory effects are exerted on the kidney, aldosterone being more potent in its mineralocorticoid effects on the kidney than is corticosterone. Release of aldosterone from the zona glomerulosa of the adrenal cortex is, in part, regulated by the peptide, angiotensin. The interrelationships between aldosterone release and sodium balance are complex. A fall in blood pressure, perhaps as a consequence of a decrease in blood volume, affects the stretch receptors in

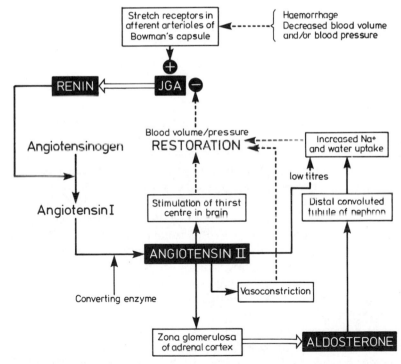

Figure 8.3   The renin-angiotensin system and the maintenance of blood volume and pressure.

the afferent arteriole of the juxtaglomerular apparatus (JGA) of the Bowman's capsule and causes the release of a proteolytic enzyme called renin: this cleaves a leucyl-leucine linkage in an α_2-globulin in the blood releasing the decapeptide angiotensin I. Angiotensin I is acted upon by converting enzyme, especially in the lungs and kidneys, where two amino acid residues are removed to produce the octapeptide angiotensin II. A third peptide, angiotensin III, which is a heptapeptide produced by aminopeptidase action on angiotension II, is also known. Angiotensins II and particularly III exert a potent action on the zona glomerulosa to release aldosterone. The target site for aldosterone is the kidney tubule, particularly the distal convoluted tubule, where it stimulates the uptake of Na^+ leading to an increased uptake of water from the collecting ducts. Thus, by increasing blood volume aldosterone helps to restore the arterial pressure to normal and, by negative feedback, prevents further release of renin (figure 8.3).

Angiotensin Angiotensin is a potent vasoconstrictor; it may play a direct role in the maintenance of blood pressure because it stimulates contraction of the heart and smooth muscle and may exert a pressor action on the vasomotor centre in the brain. Angiotensin also causes the release of ACTH and ADH from the pituitary, and catecholamines from the adrenal medulla—all of which actions may be important in indirect control of blood pressure.

Injected angiotensin stimulates a thirst centre in the diencephalon of the brain. This centre responds also to changes in the extracellular fluid volume. Stimulation by either mechanism promotes drinking and this effect of angiotensin may well be important in the hormonal control of water balance in mammals and some other vertebrates (§ 1.5).

Angiotensin may exert direct renal effects as well as those manifested through the renin-angiotensin-aldosterone system. It has been suggested that the macula densa (a region of distal tubule adjacent to the glomerulus and found only in mammals), is sentitive to distal tubule flow rates and/or sodium concentration; it may modify renin output from the juxta-glomerular granules in the afferent arteriole, to regulate GFR by controlling angiotensin levels. Administration of angiotensin, however, elicits conflicting responses, depending on the dose and on the physiological state of the animal studied. Generally, low doses are antidiuretic, high doses diuretic. This confusion may also be partly because exogenous angiotensin is received by the afferent arteriole of the glomerulus first, which may at low doses constrict and reduce GFR, whereas endogenous angiotensin may constrict the efferent arteriole to increase GFR. Without doubt, further studies are needed to clarify the direct role of angiotensin in the kidney.

8.2.2   Birds

The antidiuretic hormone in birds is vasotocin (table 1.2). Hormonal control of osmoregulation has been studied in only a few species of birds, but in ducks and fowl vasotocin increases the tubular uptake of water by increasing the permeability of the distal tubule and collecting ducts. Some nephrons in the avian kidney resemble mammalian nephrons but the others are like those of reptiles and other lower vertebrates in that they lack a hairpin-like structure. Higher doses of vasotocin reduce GFR particularly in the reptilian type of nephrons, probably by constriction of the afferent arterioles of the glomeruli. Both aldosterone and corticosterone act as they do in mammals to reduce renal loss of sodium and increase potassium secretion. Absorption of sodium and water from the coprodeum and colon is regulated partly by adrenocorticosteroids, particularly aldosterone.

In marine birds the adrenals may be involved to a greater extent in ionic regulation. Gulls living near the sea or brackish waters have larger adrenals (produce more hormone?—see §3.1.1) than those birds that drink fresh water. Whether birds possess a functional renin-angiotensin-aldosterone system is not clear; angiotensin fails to stimulate aldosterone release *in vivo* and *in vitro*. The physiological role of angiotensin in birds remains to be clarified.

Salt glands   Certain birds and reptiles possess paired glands above the orbits which discharge a fluid rich in salt; in most birds this is mainly sodium chloride, but in terrestrial herbivores like the ostrich, and marine reptiles like the iguana, which have a high dietary intake of potassium, the fluid is a variable mixture of potassium and sodium chloride. The initiation of salt gland secretion is via the parasympathetic nervous system; osmoreceptors situated either in the heart or great vessels respond to hypertonicity of the blood. The resulting vasodilation—the glands can be seen to "flush" with blood—appears to be an important aspect of salt gland function. Adrenalin, for example, inhibits the salt gland's response to hypertonic saline, probably by vasoconstrictor activity.

Fluid secretion by the salt gland begins within two minutes of an intravenous salt load; ACTH, corticosterone and prolactin each enhance secretory activity. The physiological significance of these hormonal responses of the salt gland are disputed, but it is thought that prolactin and corticosterone could have important adaptive functions during dehydration or excessive dietary salt intake respectively.

It has been suggested that the salt glands evolved as an adaptation to the needs of water retention; the reabsorption of salt and water from the coprodeum and colon is advantageous in terms of water conservation but the reabsorbed salt cannot be excreted via the kidney without further loss of water. The function of the salt glands in secreting a concentrated salt solution is thus similar to that of the gills in marine teleosts.

8.2.3 Amphibia

Phylogenetically, the amphibia were the first truly terrestrial vertebrates but they still require access to fresh water and have aquatic larvae. They thus face the problems of living in both aquatic and terrestrial environments, and their osmoregulation and its endocrine control are of considerable interest.

As a general strategy, urinary output can be reduced either by increasing tubular reabsorption or by reducing GFR. Regulation of GFR can be achieved in two ways; all nephrons may show a reduction in filtration rate, or some nephrons may cease to filter while the remainder continue—this is called *glomerular intermittency*. In contrast to the mammalian situation, where variations in urine output are largely attributable to variations in tubular reabsorption of water, amphibians show considerable variations in GFR rates. Changes in urine output correlate well with changes in GFR, suggesting that the urine volume may be adjusted by short-term changes in the number of the filtering nephrons; this may depend on the state of hydration, and be under endocrine control.

Vasotocin In amphibia the posterior pituitary contains vasotocin and mesotocin (table 1.2) but the response to these varies in different species. Vasotocin reduces GFR and increases tubular water reabsorption; this latter response, with the exception of *Necturus*, is not seen in urodeles (newts and salamanders). Decreased GFR may result from a change in renal blood flow by constriction of afferent arterioles to reduce the number of filtering nephrons. Mesotocin promotes diuresis in some anurans (frogs and toads) and in at least one urodele, by increasing GFR. Its action is not fully understood but may result from glomerular recruitment by efferent arteriole constriction.

In the aquatic toad, *Xenopus*, vasotocin is without effect upon urine flow which is perhaps to be expected because if circulating vasotocin induced water retention, the toad would become overhydrated. Indeed, survival of aquatic toads and the urodeles is probably dependent upon the loss of the water retention response. Thus young bullfrog tadpoles do not show water retention in response to vasotocin but during metamorphosis a gradual change in the kidney response occurs so that the hormone is fully effective in the adult.

Vasotocin acts also on the skin. Amphibia do not drink but they take up water across the whole surface area of their skin. In species which occupy relatively dry, rather than wet or damp habitats, vasotocin increases the permeability of the skin allowing water influx along an osmotic gradient by an action similar to that seen in the renal tubules (figure 8.4). This response to the hormone allows replacement of water lost by evaporation in dry conditions; such rehydration may be extensive, especially in species inhabiting desert areas with only sporadic access to water. The effect of vasotocin in increasing skin permeability is not seen in urodeles, nor in tadpoles or fully aquatic anura.

In many species vasotocin controls the reabsorption of water into the blood from the urinary bladder. The bladder is large and in some desert-living frogs it stores water equivalent to 50% of the body weight. Dehydration causes vasotocin to be released and in anurans, but not in most urodeles, stimulates water reabsorption from the bladder.

Adaptive radiation in amphibia is not as extensive as in other vertebrate groups but the amphibia are surprisingly diverse in the habitats they

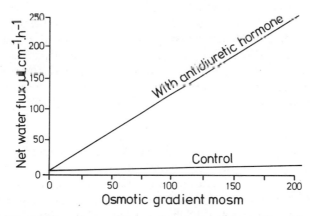

Figure 8.4 Water flux across an antidiuretic hormone-sensitive membrane (toad bladder): dependence on both the presence of hormone and the osmotic gradient between the two sides of the membrane. After Leaf, A. and Hays, R. M. (1961) *Rec. Prog. Horm. Res.*, **17**, 467–486.

occupy. For example, *Rana cancrivora* inhabits sea water mangrove swamps, and its diet of crabs is rich in salts. This frog maintains its blood plasma slightly hypertonic to the swamp water by elevating the blood levels of urea and salts so that it suffers minor osmotic flooding. The skin does not respond to vasotocin but the permeability of the bladder to urea increases in response to the hormone and allows the reabsorption of urea from the urine back into the blood.

In frog skin and bladder preparations, vasotocin stimulates Na^+ movement (in the serosal direction) but the significance of this to the overall regulation of Na^+ in the intact frog is uncertain. The major control of sodium transport at the skin and the bladder, which form part of the normal homeostasis of Na^+ levels, is exerted by aldosterone. The steroid is effective at low concentrations and is released in response to sodium depletion. It does not affect the renal reabsorption of Na^+ in amphibia, but may increase water reabsorption by controlling permeability of the tubules.

Angiotensin   The renin-angiotensin system is present in amphibians but does not appear to stimulate aldosterone production. Exogenous angiotensin has direct renal actions, but the effects are not consistent so that its renal function is uncertain; its physiological actions may be entirely extra-renal since it increases sodium uptake across the skin and increases water permeability in the bladder.

Eft drive   In some newts the terrestrial adult is called an *eft*. Injections of prolactin into efts elicit the so-called "eft drive" and cause them to seek water to breed. This eft drive can be used as a bioassay for prolactins extracted from many different vertebrates. The actions of prolactin are not fully understood but it affects the behaviour of the newt and it may also reduce the water and sodium permeability of the skin to adapt the newt to the osmotic stress of the aquatic environment (see also § 7.7.1).

8.2.4   *Teleost fishes*

Fishes represent a very diverse group which in similar environments may osmoregulate quite differently. The physiology of osmoregulation and the differences between bony fishes, elasmobranchs and jawless fish are well documented but much of the information on the role of hormones is restricted to one group of bony fish—the teleosts. Teleosts like the salmon, the trout and the eel are said to be euryhaline because they can live in both fresh water and sea water. They have attracted much interest from endocrinologists because hormones ensure the survival of these fishes in different salinities. Much of our knowledge of the roles of hormones in osmoregulation comes from studies on euryhaline species.

The pituitary gland, prolactin and cortisol　After removal of the pituitary gland, both fresh water and marine teleosts show a general tendency towards osmotic and ionic equilibration with the environment. Hence, in fresh water, the blood osmolarity decreases due to osmotic entry of water, its sodium and chloride content decreases, and tissue water increases. In sea water, hypophysectomized teleosts have increased plasma osmolarity and tissue dehydration. These effects could represent a total endocrine deficiency leading to physiological collapse, but it is now realized that rather specific lesions are responsible for the effects of hypophysectomy on osmoregulation; they result directly from a lack of prolactin, and indirectly from a lack of cortisol due to removal of ACTH producing cells in the pituitary. The effects of removal of the pituitary vary between species and between fish living in fresh or salt water. For example, the fresh water teleost *Poecilia* dies in fresh water soon after hypophysectomy unless injected with prolactin. Similarly, after hypophysectomy the marine killifish, *Fundulus*, osmoregulates in sea water but soon dies in fresh water unless given prolactin; no other hormones have this effect. Some fresh water teleosts like the goldfish, the trout and the eel can survive hypophysectomy for considerable periods, although hypophysectomized eels, for example, cannot osmoregulate when transferred to sea water unless they are injected with ACTH or cortisol.

It is now generally accepted that prolactin and cortisol are the two major hormones concerned with osmoregulation in teleosts; cortisol predominates in sea water and prolactin in fresh water adaptation. These two hormones act on all the osmoregulatory organs—the gills, intestine, kidney and urinary bladder (figure 8.5). Cortisol stimulates drinking behaviour in marine teleosts and acts on epithelia in the osmoregulatory organs to increase absorption or excretion of Na^+ and Cl^- by stimulating ion pumps; in most cases membrane permeability to water also increases. The responses to cortisol are usually slow, with a latency of a few hours, but are long-lived. It is interesting that cortisol acts in these ways as a mineralocorticoid in teleosts—its effects in tetrapods are primarily upon intermediary metabolism. Aldosterone has only been demonstrated in a few teleost species, and cortisol may therefore fulfill the roles of both a mineralo- and a glucocorticoid hormone.

The primary action of prolactin is probably to reduce membrane

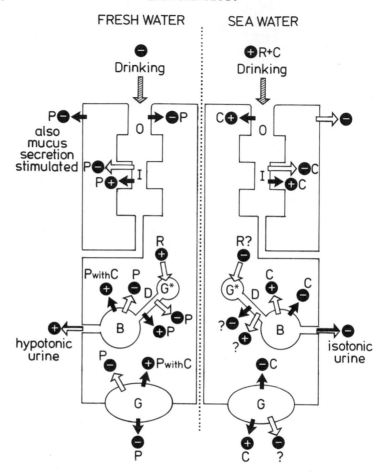

Figure 8.5 Schematic illustration of the hormonal control of salt and water balance in fresh water and sea water teleosts. G = gill; B = bladder; G* = glomerulus; I = intestine; O = oesophagus; D = distal tubule; R = renin-angiotensin system; C = cortisol; P = prolactin. The solid and open arrows represent sodium and water movement respectively.

permeability to ions and water but its actions on many ion-transporting epithelia interact with those of cortisol and other hormones. Thus although cortisol appears to be the principal sea water adaptation hormone, it is important in salt conservation for fresh water teleosts and acts synergistically with prolactin to·activate sodium pumps in the bladder, the kidney, and the gills. In its effects on reducing membrane permeability, however, prolactin opposes the effects of cortisol (figure 8.5).

In the eel, adaptation from fresh water to sea water involves a complete replacement of the oesophageal epithelium which is known to contribute to osmoregulation. The oesophageal wall changes from a stratified epithelium rich in mucus cells to a simple columnar epithelium. It is not certain whether prolactin and/or cortisol control this cellular reorganization but both hormones affect the permeability of the oesophageal epithelium; cortisol increases, while prolactin decreases membrane permeability to ions (the impermeability of the oesophagus to water is unaffected by either hormone). It is suggested that in sea water eels, ingested sea water is desalted before it enters the intestine so that absorption of water takes place without loss of water from the body.

Vasotocin Vasotocin may be involved in osmoregulation in teleosts. Exogenous hormone exerts antidiuretic effects in the lake and rainbow trout, but in the goldfish it is diuretic. In fresh water eels the response is dose-dependent; large doses are diuretic, but small amounts antidiuretic. These diuretic and antidiuretic responses probably result solely from alteration in total GFR; they possibly involve recruitment of previously non-filtering nephrons to give diuretic responses, or a reduction in the number of filtering nephrons to give antidiuretic responses.

A further action of vasotocin might be in controlling ion exchange at the gills. It might affect gill permeability in a manner analogous to the action of neurohypophysial peptides in tetrapods but it is more likely that the vasoactive properties of vasotocin produce localized changes in the blood distribution within the gill to alter ion transfer. Adrenalin decreases salt excretion and increases water uptake across the gills and it has been argued that adrenalin and vasotocin could exert short term changes in the gill function indirectly by haemodynamic actions (it is now known, however, that adrenalin acts directly on the water permeability and chloride secretion in the gill). Recently vasotocin has been found in the blood of fishes at sufficiently high titres (measured by RIA) to suggest that its pressor effects could be of physiological significance.

The renin-angiotensin system Renal renin activity and juxtoglomerular cells are found in teleosts but their physiological role is uncertain. In the toadfish, *Opsanus*, haemorrhage causes an increase in plasma renin within 30 min, suggesting that angiotensin may be involved in the regulation of blood pressure in teleosts, as it is in birds and mammals. Injected mammalian angiotensin has potent pressor activity in fishes but other actions of the hormone may be quite different from those seen in mammals. For example, aldosterone synthesis appears not to be a general capability of teleosts and is therefore not a likely target for angiotensin. Indeed, there is no clear evidence to suggest that the renin-angiotensin system is activated and helps to conserve sodium in sodium-depleted teleosts. Fish angiotensins may, however, be concerned with osmo-regulation by acting on the kidney to control GFR.

In the trout, for example, glomerular intermittency is markedly influ-enced by infusion of angiotensin. In fresh water trout the hormone has no effect on GFR in individual nephrons but it decreases urine production by reducing dramatically the number of filtering nephrons to resemble the situation observed in the sea water adapted trout. This suggests that the renin-angiotensin system may play a key role in adaptation to hyper-osmotic media by regulating the patterns of blood flow within the kidney (and by stimulating drinking behaviour; § 1.5). In the eel, however, exogenous angiotensins increase GFR. This confusing situation is remin-iscent of that in the amphibia but the contradictory results may be due to species differences and in the actions of endogenous and exogenous angiotensins.

The urophysis and corpuscles of Stannius   These structures are endocrine-like in appearance and appear to show changes in cellular activity in different osmotic conditions. Although surgical removal leads to deficiences in osmoregulatory ability, and extracts of the tissues alter the balance of water and electrolytes, a major physiological role in osmo-regulation is uncertain for either endocrine centre. The evidence at present suggests that the corpuscles of Stannius play a minor role in osmo-regulation by their actions on calcium metabolism (§ 6.3.2).

BIBLIOGRAPHY

The reader's attention is also drawn to the references given in many of the figure legends.

General reading
Bentley, P. J. (1976) *Comparative Vertebrate Endocrinology*, C.U.P.
"Calcium and cell regulation" (1974) *Biochem. Soc. Symp.*, No. 39 (R. M. S. Smellie, ed.) Biochem. Soc., London.
"Calcium in biological systems" (1976) *Symposia of the S.E.B.*, No. XXX (C. J. Duncan, ed.), C.U.P.
Denton, R. M. and Pogson, C. I. (1976) *Metabolic regulation*, Chapman and Hall, London.
Finean, J. B., Coleman, R. and Michell, R. H. (1978) *Membranes and their Cellular Functions* (2nd edition) Blackwell Scientific Publications, Oxford.
Gaillard, P. J. and Boer, H. H. (1978) *Comparative Endocrinology*, Elsevier/North Holland.
Highnam, K. C. and Hill, L. (1977) *The Comparative Endocrinology of the Invertebrates* (2nd edition) Edward Arnold.
Invertebrate Neurosecretion (1976). *American Zoologist*, **16**, No. 2, 103–271.
Maddrell, S. H. P. and Nordmann, J. J. (1979) *Neurosecretion*, Blackie & Son Ltd.
Methods in Enzymology (1975) Vols. XXXVI to XL, "Hormone action and related methodology" (B. W. O'Malley and J. G. Hardman, eds.) Academic Press, New York.
Peptide Hormones (1976) (J. A. Parsons, ed.) Macmillan Press.
The Juvenile Hormones (1976) (L. I. Gilbert, ed.) Plenum Press.

Chapter 1
Brownstein, M. J. (1977) "Biologically active peptides in the mammalian central nervous system", in *Peptides in Neurobiology* (H. Gainer, ed.) 145–170, Plenum Press.
Elde, R. and Hökfelt, T. (1979) "Localization of hypophysiotropic peptides and other biologically active peptides within the brain", *Ann. Rev. Physiol.*, **41**, 587–602.
Guillemin, R. (1976) "The expanding significance of hypothalamic peptides, or, Is endocrinology a branch of neuroendocrinology?" *Rec. Prog. Horm. Res.*, **33**, 1–28.
Klee, W. A. (1977) "Endogenous opiate peptides", in *Peptides in Neurobiology* (H. Gainer, ed.) 375–396, Plenum Press.
Pearse, A. G. E. (1976) "Peptides in brain and intestine", *Nature*, **262**, 92–94.
Shire, J. G. M. (1976) "The forms, uses and significance of genetic variation in endocrine systems", *Biol. Rev.*, **51**, 105–141.
Wallis, M. (1975) "The molecular evolution of pituitary hormones", *Biol. Rev.*, **50**, 35–98.
Vale, W. *et al.*, (1977) "Regulatory peptides of the hypothalamus", *Ann. Rev. Physiol.*, **39**, 473–527.

Chapter 2

Berlind, A. (1977) "Cellular dynamics in invertebrate neurosecretory systems", *Int. Rev. Cytology*, **49**, 171–251.

Christensen, A. K. and Gillim, S. W. (1969) "The correlation of fine structure and function in steroid-secreting cells with emphasis on those of the gonads", in *The Gonads* (K. W. McKerns, ed.) 415–488, North Holland Publ. Co., Amsterdam.

Cooke, I. M. (1977) "Electrical activity of neurosecretory terminals and control of peptide hormone release", in *Peptides in Neurobiology* (H. Gainer, ed.) 345–374, Plenum Press.

Cross, B. A. *et al.*, (1974) "Endocrine Neurons", *Rec. Prog. Horm. Res.*, **31**, 243–294.

Dahl, G. *et al.*, (1979) "Models for exocytotic membrane fusion", in *Secretory Mechanisms* (C. R. Hopkins and C. J. Duncan, eds.) 349–368. *Symposia of the S.E.B.*, No. XXXIII, C.U.P.

Fawcett, D. W. *et al.*, (1969) "The ultrastructure of endocrine glands", *Rec. Progr. Horm. Res.*, **25**, 315–380.

Frontali, N. and Gainer, H. (1977) "Peptides in invertebrate nervous systems", in *Peptides in Neurobiology* (H. Gainer, ed.) 259–294, Plenum Press.

Kern, H. F. *et al.*, (1979) "Regulation of intracellular transport of exportable proteins in the rat exocrine pancreas", in *Secretory Mechanisms* (C. R. Hopkins and C. J. Duncan, eds.) 79–99, *Symposia of the S.E.B.*, No. XXXIII, C.U.P.

Lands, W. E. M. (1979) "The biosynthesis and metabolism of prostaglandins", *Ann. Rev. Physiol.*, **41**, 633–652.

Marks, N. (1977) "Conversion and inactivation of neuropeptides", in *Peptides in Neurobiology* (H. Gainer, ed.) 221–258, Plenum Press.

Normann, T. C. (1978) "Neurosecretion by exocytosis", *Int. Rev. Cytology*, **53**, 1–77.

Salvatore, G. and Edelhoch, H. (1973) "Chemistry and biosynthesis of thyroid iodoproteins", in *Hormonal Proteins and Peptides*, Vol. 1 (C. Hao Li, ed) 201–241, Academic Press.

Samuelsson, B. (1977) "Prostaglandins and thromboxanes", *Rec. Prog. Horm. Res.*, **34**, 239–258.

Sief, S. M. and Robinson, A. G. (1978) "Localization and release of neurophysins", *Ann. Rev. Physiol.*, **40**, 345–376.

Chapter 3

Gilbert, L. I. *et al.*, (1978) "Regulation of juvenile hormone titre in Lepidoptera", in *Comparative Endocrinology* (P. J. Gaillard and H. H. Boer, eds.) 471–486, Elsevier/North Holland Biomedical Press, Amsterdam.

Koolman, J. (1978) "Metabolism of ecdysteroids", in *Comparative Endocrinology* (P. J. Gaillard and H. H. Boer, eds.) 495–498, Elsevier/North Holland Biomedical Press, Amsterdam.

Methods of Hormone Radioimmunoassay (1979) (2nd edition) (B. M. Jaffe and H. R. Behrman, eds.) Academic Press, New York.

Straus, E. and Yalow, R. S. (1977) "Specific problems in the identification and quantitation of neuropeptides by radioimmunoassay", in *Peptides in Neurobiology* (H. Gainer, ed.) 31–60, Plenum Press.

Tait, J. F. and Burstein, S. (1964) "*In vivo* studies of steroid dynamics in man", in *The Hormones*, Vol. V (G. Pincus and K. V. Thimann, eds.) 441–557, Academic Press, New York.

Chapter 4

Avery, A. S. *et al.*, (1966) "Protein-steroid interactions and their role in the transport and metabolism of steroids", in *Steroid Dynamics* (G. Pincus, T. Nakao and J. F. Tait, eds.) 1–61, Academic Press, New York.

Baxter, J. D. *et al.*, (1979) "Thyroid hormone receptors and responses", *Rec. Prog. Horm. Res.*, **35**, 97–153.

Cohen, P. (1976) *Control of Enzyme Activity*, Chapman and Hall.

"Hormone Receptors" (1978) (D. M. Klachko, L. R. Forte and J. M. Franz, eds.) *Advances in Experimental Medicine and Biology*, **96**, Plenum Press.

O'Malley, B. W. O. *et al.*, (1979) "The ovalbumin gene: organization, structure, transcription and regulation", *Rec. Prog. Horm. Res.*, **35**, 1–46.

Rasmussen, H. *et al.*, (1979) "The messenger function of calcium in cell activation", in *Secretory Mechanisms* (C. R. Hopkins and C. J. Duncan, eds.) 161–197, *Symposia of the S.E.B.*, No. XXXIII, C.U.P.

Receptors and Hormone Action, Vol. III (1978) (L. Birnbaumer and B. W. O'Malley, eds.) Academic Press.

Reproduction in Mammals, Book 7 (1979) "Mechanisms of hormone action" (C. R. Austin and R. V. Short, eds.) C.U.P.

Robison, G. A., Butcher, R. W. and Sutherland, E. W. (1971) *Cyclic AMP*, Academic Press, New York.

Weller, M. (1979) *Protein Phosphorylation*, Pion Limited.

Chapter 5

Bailey, E. (1975) "Biochemistry of insect flight, part 2, fuel supply", in *Insect Biochemistry and Function* (D. J. Candy and B. A. Kilby, eds.) 88–176, Chapman and Hall.

Crabtree, B. and Newsholme, E. A. (1975) "Comparative aspects of fuel utilization and metabolism by muscle", in *Insect Muscle* (P. N. R. Usherwood, ed.) 405–500, Academic Press.

Dockray, G. J. (1979) "Comparative biochemistry and physiology of gut hormones", *Ann. Rev. Physiol.*, **41**, 83–95.

Felig, P. *et al.*, (1979) "Hormonal interactions in the regulation of blood glucose", *Rec. Prog. Horm. Res.*, **35**, 501–532.

Jagannadha Rao, A. and Ramachandran, J. (1977) "Growth hormone and the regulation of lipolysis", in *Hormonal Proteins and Peptides*, Vol. IV (C. Hao Li, ed.) 43–60, Academic Press, New York.

Johnson, L. R. (1977) "Gastrointestinal hormones and their functions", *Ann. Rev. Physiol.*, **39**, 135–158.

Masoro, E. J. (1977) "Lipids and lipid metabolism", *Ann. Rev. Physiol.*, **39**, 301–321.

Newsholme, E. A. and Start, C. (1974) *Regulation in Metabolism* (2nd edition), John Wiley and Sons.

"Regulatory mechanisms of carbohydrate metabolism" (1977) (V. Esmann, ed.) FEBS, 11th meeting, Copenhagen, Pergamon Press, 42, No. A1.

Steele, J. E. (1976) "Hormonal control of metabolism in insects", *Adv. Insect Physiol.*, **12**, 239–323.

Trygstad, O. (1977) "Growth hormone, biochemical aspects", in *Growth Factors*, FEBS, 11th meeting, Copenhagen, (K. W. Kastrup and J. H. Nielson, eds.) 85–94, Pergamon Press

Unger, R. H. and Dobbs, R. E. (1978) "Insulin, glucagon and somatostatin secretion in the regulation of metabolism", *Ann. Rev. Physiol.*, **40**, 307–343.

Chapter 6

"Calcium-regulating hormones" (1975) (R. V. Talmage, M. Owen and J. A. Parsons, eds.) *Excerpta Medica*.

"Comparative biology of skin" (1975) (R. I. C. Spearman, ed.) *Symposia of the Zoological Society of London*, No. 39, Academic Press.

Geschwind, I. I. *et al.*, (1972) "The effect of melanocyte-stimulating hormone on coat color in the mouse", *Rec. Prog. Horm. Res.*, **28**, 91–130.

Jungreis, A. M. (1979) "Physiology of moulting in insects", *Adv. Insect. Physiol.*, **14**, 109–183.

"Melanocyte stimulating hormone: control, chemistry and effects" (1977) (F. J. H. Tilders, D. F. Swaab and TJ. B. van Wimersma Greidanus), S. Karger.

Rees, H. H. (1977) *Insect Biochemistry*, Chapman and Hall.

Richards, A. G. (1978) "The chemistry of insect cuticle" in *Biochemistry of Insects* (M. Rockstein, ed.) 205–232, Academic Press.

Chapter 7

Behrman, (1979) "Prostaglandins in hypothalamo-pituitary and ovarian function", *Ann. Rev. Physiol.*, **41**, 685–700.

Barker Jørgensen, C. (1974) "Integrative functions of the brain", in *Physiology of the Amphibia*, Vol. II (B. Lofts, ed.) 1–51, Academic Press.

Dorrington, J. H. and Armstrong, D. T. (1979) "Effects of FSH on gonadal functions", *Rec. Prog. Horm. Res.*, **35**, 301–342.

Engelemann, F. (1979) "Insect vitellogenin: identification, biosynthesis and role in vitellogenesis", *Adv. Insect Physiol.*, **14**, 49–108.

Etkin, W. (1970) "The endocrine mechanism of amphibian metamorphosis, an evolutionary achievement", in *Hormones and the Environment, Memoirs of the Society for Endocrinology*, **18** (G. K. Benson and J. G. Phillips, eds.) 137–155, C.U.P.

Fink, G. (1979) "Neuroendocrine control of gonadotrophin secretion", *Brit. Med. Bull.*, **35**(2), 155–160.

Golding, D. W. (1974) "A survey of neuroendocrine phenomena in non-arthropod invertebrates", *Biol. Rev.*, **49**, 161–224.

Heap, R. B. *et al.*, (1979) "Role of embryonic signals in the establishment of pregnancy", *Brit. Med. Bull.*, **35**(2), 129–135.

Henderson, K. M. (1979) "Gonadotrophic regulation of ovarian activity", *Brit. Med. Bull.*, **35**(2), 161–166.

Krulich, L. (1979) "Central neurotransmitters and the secretion of prolactin, GH, LH and TSH", *Ann. Rev. Physiol.*, **41**, 603–615.

Labrie, F. *et al.*, (1979) "Mechanism of action of hypothalamic hormones in the adenohypophysis", *Ann. Rev. Physiol.*, **41**, 555–569.

Liggins, G. C. (1979) "Initiation of parturition", *Brit. Med. Bull.*, **35**(2), 145–150.

Mordue, W. *et al.*, (1980) *Insect Physiology*, Blackwell Scientific Publications, Oxford.

Richards, J. S. (1979) "Hormonal control of ovarian follicular development: A 1978 perspective", *Rec. Prog. Horm. Res.*, **35**, 343–373.

Salthe, S. N. and Mecham, J. S. (1974) "Reproductive and courtship patterns", in *Physiology of the Amphibia*, Vol. II (B. Lofts, ed.) 309–521, Academic Press.

Schally, A. V. *et al.*, (1978) "Hypothalamic regulatory hormones", *Ann. Rev. Biochem.*, **47**, 89–128.

Chapter 8

Bentley, P. J. (1971) *Endocrines and Osmoregulation: a comparative account of the regulation of water and salt in vertebrates*, Springer-Verlag, Berlin.

Hirano, T. *et al.*, (1978) "Angiotensin and drinking in the eel and the frog", in *Osmotic and Volume Regulation*, Alfred Benzon Symposium XI (C. Barker Jørgensen and E. Skadhauge, eds.) 122–134, Munksgaard, Copenhagen.

Johnson, D. W. (1973) "Endocrine control of hydromineral balance in teleosts", *Amer. Zool.*, **13**, 799–818.

Katz, A. I. and Lindheimer, M. D. (1977) "Actions of hormones on the kidney", *Ann. Rev. Physiol.*, **39**, 109–183.

Maetz, J., Payan, P. and de Renzis, G. (1976) "Controversial aspects of ionic uptake in fresh water animals", in *Perspectives in Experimental Biology*, Vol. 1 (P. Spencer Davis, ed.) 77–92, Pergamon Press.

Nishimura, H. (1978) "Physiological evolution of the renin-angiotensin system", *Jap. Heart J.*, **19**, 806–822.

Peaker, M. and Linzell, J. L. (1975) "Salt glands in birds and reptiles", *Monographs of the Physiological Society*, No. 32, C.U.P.

Reid, I. A. *et al.*, (1978) "The renin-angiotensin system", *Ann. Rev. Physiol.*, **40**, 377–410.
Shoemaker, V. H. (1977) "Osmoregulation in amphibians and reptiles", *Ann. Rev. Physiol.*, **39**, 449–471.
Sokabe, H. (1974) "Phylogeny of the renal effects of angiotensin", *Kidney Int.*, **6**, 263–271.
Skadhauge, E. and Maloiy, G. M. O. (1978) "The intestine and osmoregulation" in *Osmotic and Volume Regulation*, Alfred Benzon Symposium XI (C. Barker Jørgensen and E. Skadhauge, eds.) 325–343, Munksgaard, Copenhagen.

POSTSCRIPT TO BIBLIOGRAPHY

Hormones and Evolution (1980) Vols. 1 and 2. (E. J. W. Barrington, ed.) Academic Press, London.
Hormones in Blood (1979) 3rd edition, Vols. 1, 2 and 3. (C. H. Gray and V. H. T. James, eds.) Academic Press, London.
Neurohormonal Techniques in Insects (1980). (T. A. Miller, ed.) Springer-Verlag, New York.

INDEX

179